THE GRAY ITCH

THE

Also by Edmond Hallberg

When I Was Your Age (with William Thomas)

GRAY ITCH

The Male Metapause Syndrome

EDMOND C. HALLBERG

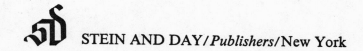

STEIN AND DAY/*Publishers*/New York

First Stein and Day edition 1978
Copyright © 1977 by Ombudsman Press
Copyright © 1978 by Edmond C. Hallberg
A limited number of copies of an earlier edition of this work were
privately published by the author under the title *The Grey Itch.*
All rights reserved
Designed by Ed Kaplin
Printed in the United States of America
Stein and Day/*Publishers*/ Scarborough House,
Briarcliff Manor, N.Y. 10510

Library of Congress Cataloging in Publication Data

Hallberg, Edmond C.
    The gray itch.

    Privately published in 1977 under title: The grey
itch.
    Bibliography: p. 209
    Includes index.
    1. Climacteric, Male.   I. Title.
RC884.H3   1978   612.6′65   77-92713
ISBN 0-8128-2439-3

To
Kaylene

ACKNOWLEDGMENTS

Many people contributed to this book: college youths, middle-aged men, and the female partners of metapausal men attempting to understand the "strange foreigners" their husbands had become. Buses, bars, and barbershops were often fruitful settings to talk of mid-life.

Any attempt to describe a new set of conditions requires the thought of many, most of whom are not related to the scientific world, each attempting to paint a picture of the metapausal man.

My thanks go to those men in our middle-aged mens' groups at CSULA and those with whom I counseled after the aerospace crash in Los Angeles in 1972. The willingness of many to cross the traditional "male silence barrier" and talk of their problems in mid-life was most important in moving this book to fruition.

Equally, important were the thoughts of others with whom I counseled; some quietly in the corner of a room during a cocktail party; others in my office. Each brought new concerns and interests to the subject and forced me beyond my own initial thinking.

Beyond these many, special thanks must be given to those who worked directly in the formulation of this book.

Thanks should be given to my colleagues who stretched and pulled at "Male Metapause" as a concept: Herb Levitt, Len Steinberg, Curly Johnson, Bill Thomas, and Ursala Vils of the *Los Angeles Times*.

Special thanks go to Jeff and Kathy Cohen, who offered constructive criticism, research, editing, typing, and personal support. Jeff's ability to effectively coin words such as "metacare" added greatly to the new vocabulary of metapause and metathought.

viii ACKNOWLEDGMENTS

Appreciation is also extended to Luther Nicholes, West Coast editor of Doubleday, Inc. Luther's interest and openness were greatly appreciated in a day when a lack of interest or a brief polite comment represent the only commentary many publishers feel they can afford to make.

Thanks to buddies like J. McCuen, J. Flood, W. Thomas, B. Martin, and B. Nixon for their initial perusal and criticism.

Special appreciation to Kristen and Karin Hallberg for their love and their understanding during my time away, and of a father who "just had to write this book." This was particularly appreciated inasmuch as it was a time when we needed each other the most.

Sandra Phelps' editing and comments would have made my freshman English teacher very happy. Her intelligent questions and skill in editing added greatly to the clarity and completeness of this work.

Many others who typed and Xeroxed early segments should be recognized. Kathy Lee, Judy Clements, and Judy Grutter need particular mention. Also, thanks to Bill Gehr and his staff at the Trident Bookstore, and especially Peggy Friberg. Their support was crucial to this publication. Appreciation must also go to Jim and Evelyn Shupe for their hospitality at Laguna Beach.

Lastly, special appeciation goes to Kaylene, who patiently listened to me form, discard, and reform thoughts and concepts. Her helpful criticism and encouragement indicated a quiet faith beyond her personal and professional support. This faith was a continuing source of enlightenment. In appreciation, this book is dedicated to her.

E.C.H.

Contents

Part I

IS THAT ALL THERE IS?

Life is action and passion: Therefore, it is required of a man that he should share the passion and action of his time at the peril of being judged not to have lived.
—OLIVER WENDELL HOLMES

Chapter 1

LEFT TURN AT OAK STREET?

Having trouble climbing a tree with your kids? Tempted more by your secretary's legs than your boss's income? Going for bigger checks in your sportscoats? Given up pulling out those gray hairs for fear of premature baldness? If this is you, these represent the first traces of a barrage of meteorlike metathoughts that rock the male spaceship on its rendezvous with ages thirty-five to fifty-five.

This book is in response to these questions and an old one: "Why do middle-aged men start acting so differently?" "Why would a happily married man suddenly announce he's going to climb Mt. Everest or buy a Maserati?" "Why would an excellent engineer turn down a fine aerospace position when he has been out of work for three months?" "Why would fat old George perform the bump and fondle his way through half the women under thirty at a neighbor's party?" Male metapause may be the reason.

Male metapause represents an important life stage. Unlike the menopause of the female, however, the outward changes of metapause in the male are subtle, small, and sometimes unnoticed. A panicked questioning occurs in males during this time. A flickering concern illuminates this mid-life condition. "Who am I?" and "Where am I going?" are constant questions.

I've been seriously searching for answers to these questions for the past five years. During the 1970 aerospace layoffs, I was contracted to assist one hundred of those "let go" to "get hold

3

of themselves" and find new employment in mid-life. Throughout the counseling seminars, the recurring theme was not "Where do I find work?" but "Who am I—now that I'm forty-five?" The symptoms of metapause described in this book surfaced as the hidden agenda in these early group-counseling sessions.

Male Metapause

The word *metapause,* found in these pages, should be taken literally: *meta* means a change in form. Metapause relates as in metaphysics, the nature of existence—"Who am I?" It means, as in metacenter, an intersection of vertical lines. The intersection is mid-life.

Statements such as "I'm not going to be president of the company" or "The kids don't need me anymore" are a result of the "pause" in metapause. These pauses lead to thoughts that occur while one drives to work, gets into bed, or burns the midnight oil at Amalgamated. Metapausal thoughts—meta-thoughts—are well depicted by Roy Clark's song "Right or Left on Oak Street":

> The alarm rang at seven this morning,
> the same time it did yesterday.
> Seven-thirty is my breakfast time,
> and I know what the wife's gonna say.
>
> Crawford's next door got a new swimmin' pool,
> the Miller's got a color T.V.
> Mr. Wilson's job is not as good as yours,
> but his wife dresses better'n me.
>
> I get to school at 8:05
> and drop the kids off at a gate.
> I drive past the clock outside the bank,
> and it's exactly a quarter past eight.
>
> When I reach the stop sign at Oak Street
> the same thought crosses my mind:

Should I turn right as I always have
or left and leave it all behind?

Right or left at Oak Street—
the choice I face every day.
And I don't know which takes more courage ...
the stayin' or the runnin' away.[1]

The metathought: "Should I turn right or left at Oak Street?"
Waiting at the stop sign at Oak Street does represent the *pause*
in metapause: These thoughts, the first questions of "Who am
I?," are pushed into subconsciousness by that honking line of
neighbors behind us. And we go on, only to have a new
metathought appear again when we least expect it.

These pauses between youth and old age bring to focus the
greater preoccupations of *metapause,* questions of "being," of
existence, of me.

Metapause is also so subtle and private that the victim, his
family, fellow golfers, and occasional girl friends sometimes
don't even recognize it. Loneliness is often with us.

Being alone is set against these roller coaster highs of life: a
romance, occasional closeness at home, and shooting 79 on the
golf course. Through all of these ups and downs, the "Who am
I?" seems to persist as a private matter, like a cold you can't
shake or a bill you never quite pay off.

We men are notorious, aren't we, for keeping these highs and
lows to ourselves—as if silence were a sign of machismo. Men
don't talk about "Who am I?" Only women worry about
themselves. We say, "Oh, nothing," when asked what's wrong
by a wife or colleague—and in our loneliness, we struggle alone.

If metapause is happening to you, read on. You don't need to
"tough it out" alone. It doesn't have to be like discovering,
weeks later, that you and all your fraternity brothers got that
social disease from the nice little sorority girl, yet nobody's
mentioning it. If you say you're not full of metathoughts, either
you're kidding yourself or you should sell the book to a friend
for half price and possibly save a career, a marriage, or forty-
year-old all ready to "find himself" in Aspen.

Meta has another meaning—that which refers to moving on beyond the questions. Throughout metapause we struggle to see ourselves, constantly wiping our sleeves in circles on the foggy mirror of "Who am I?" As we work at it, we get a new glance at ourselves; a new me does appear. At first we appear a little more wrinkled, but it is me. We are approaching Meta +. The pause has been only temporary.

Meta + isn't an uninhabited planet. It is a time of life full of adventure, influence, and caring; and it is now. It is a time to captain our own ship, make our claim, become our own power source. It becomes a time for new direction, for new careers, for knowing "me"—maybe for the first time. Meta + is a time of coupling maximum experience and influence in corporate and familial matters with the heights of our emotional maturity.

This guidance system through mid-life from metapause to emansumated man should help. The navigational points included in this book are the result of countless hours of listening to friends' stories over the bar, group and individual counseling sessions, research and personal experience.

Today, at California State University at Los Angeles, groups are being conducted for men from all walks of life, as is counseling for women who wish to understand metapause in their graying partners. Emerging from these counselees have been deep existential questions of loneliness, death, happiness, as well as some of the best barroom humor.

Within these pages we face The Gray Itch straight on as a time of crisis, analyze why the crisis has occurred, look at turning right or left at Oak Street, and offer some ways of focusing on ourselves for the road ahead.

Before you start the book, laugh at yourself. If you feel sorry for yourself or have a "poor-me" attitude, think of four things you have done in recent months that typify your middle age and are amusing to you, such as going to a discotheque and asking an eighteen-year-old to dance, or taking off for parts unknown in the mountains, or not returning to that important meeting after lunch.

If you have trouble laughing, think of the following birthday celebration, related by a California business executive:

Two weeks ago was my forty-fifth birthday. I went in to breakfast knowing that my wife would be pleasant and say "Happy birthday" and have a present for me. But she didn't even say "Good morning," let alone "Happy birthday."

I said to myself, "Well, that's a wife for you. The children will remember." The children came in to breakfast and didn't say a word.

As I walked into my office, my secretary, Janet, said, "Good morning, Boss—happy birthday," and I felt better—*someone* had remembered.

I worked until noon. About noon, Janet said, "It's your birthday, let's go to lunch, just you and me." I said, "By George, that is the greatest thing I have heard all day. Let's go."

We went out into the country to a little private place. We had two martinis and enjoyed lunch tremendously.

On the way back to the office, she said, "You know, it's such a beautiful day, we don't need to go back to the office, do we?" I said, "No, I guess not." She said, "Let's go by my apartment and I'll fix you another martini." We went to her apartment. She said, "Boss, if you don't mind, I'll go into my bedroom and slip into something more comfortable," and I told her I didn't mind at all (wow!).

She went into the bedroom and then came out carrying a big birthday cake, followed by my wife and children. All were singing "Happy Birthday," and there I sat with nothing on but my socks.

So, laughing at yourself is important.

Secondly, if you think you're the only one going through metapause, have a fellow sufferer punch your card. We don't need any martyrs. Group counseling has shown many similarities in the experiences of middle-aged men.

Third, the book is not designed to get you off the hook by saying, "It's all your wife's fault." It is written so that the average guy from thirty-five to fifty-five will get it straight that his problems are due partly to his age, time and place and are his own responsibility. It is hoped this understanding of the causes and characteristics of The Gray Itch can give you a new definition of *macho*—power over your life.

This book is divided into three parts. Part I, "Is That All There Is?," represents a description of the man and his forty-year-old male metapause syndrome, his new needs, his bizarre behavior, his yo-yo high and low reactions. The first chapters develop the idea that The Gray Itch is, in fact, a "Who am I?" identity crisis for the middle-aged man. We look at our total life cycle for a better understanding of where we are today.

At issue in Part II, "Let Me Out of Here," are the elements of who we are and where we are going in our mid-life. In the past, we determined who we were by our physical selves, our careers, our families, our wives, kids, and sex lives.

In mid-life, all of these people, places, and things—the anchors and mirrors of our identities—change, leaving us stranded in ourselves, estranged in aging bodies, not being our own best friend.

In Part III, "We Only Go Around Once," we develop a sense of centering or refocusing. We analyze where we are and would like to be through the results of a survey entitled the Hallberg Index of Male Metapause (H.I.M.M.). Based on the index scores, we select metacare action plans to gather power over ourselves and develop strategies for our future. This process helps us to center on our real selves, which in turn gives us the green light to again relate to others, to turn right or left on Oak Street.

Chapter 2

THE MALE METAPAUSE SYNDROME

We are the American middle-aged males, a minority of our population, yet the largest payers of individual income tax, the men who carry the greatest corporate and familial responsibilities of our gender—and we are in trouble.

We feel different from the way we did when we were twenty. Metathoughts—"I'm tired of my work" and "What am I going to do with the rest of my life?"—leave us wondering. We really aren't too sure of who or what we are. Our trouble stems from our changing mid-life identity. We look into the mirror and feel estranged at home and at work.

Characteristics of The Gray Itch, the male metapause, do not have universal symptoms, as acne does.

The mirrors of the male metapause syndrome, the benchmarks, are in ourselves. It's reflected by the kids, the wife, the bills, or the boss, but *it's us*. We are changing, changing what we believe in, what we look like, what we wish to be. And what we are is directly related to how we act and behave.

These changes in us are often unnoticed—for a while. Then, suddenly, as we are driving or looking into a mirror, we are different. We are into the male metapause syndrome, The Gray Itch. Take Jim's metapausal discovery. Jim was in one of the local "watering holes" between his office and home with a friend.

"... Another Friday night," Jim moaned.

"Yeah," his friend said. "What are you going to do on the big weekend?"

"Oh, I don't know ... screw around. Donna [Jim's wife] has invited over our new neighbors for dinner tonight."

"Sounds like fun."

"Bullshit, another lady-talk evening. I get loaded and they bullshit! What I need is some excitement—maybe a cute little blonde. ... Particularly after the week I've had."

"Why?" his friend said. "What's so different about this week?"

"Well, it's been one of the worst weeks of my life. I'm changing and it's scaring the hell out of me. It all started Monday when George, my sales partner, died. You know George, he lived over on Chatby."

"Yeah."

"Well, George was my partner for eight years. He sold the computers and I worked with the customers. George sat right next to me, at his desk ... right next to me. He fell right over ... and only forty-seven years old. Can you imagine, forty-seven years old ... and dead ... I can't believe it! We had old George's funeral Tuesday.

"Then, Wednesday morning," Jim continued, "I looked at myself in the mirror, in a different way, while shaving. I think that one look aged me ... aged me ten years."

"Oh, sure," his friend said. "You're really an old man at thirty-nine."

"Well, let me tell you the rest of it," Jim interrupted. "As I looked at myself in the mirror, I really studied my face, and there I was, vice-president of Amalgamated—but that's all I'm ever going to be in the company! I looked healthy, but I'm losing my sex appeal. My time is limited. I'm getting to be an old bastard! I only have so much time left. What a feeling!

"Then, I started thinking about doing something different. I started thinking about Gauguin. What a guy, dropping out of the Paris banking scene and taking off for the South Seas.

"So I took a long lunch and walked around town. I caught myself stopping at store windows, all of which were travel offices or liquor stores. It seems I either wanted to get the hell out or drown my sorrows. What do you think of that? Furthermore, all I could see as I walked were legs and tits. Girl after girl after girl ... like a ten-year-old in a candy store. 'What's the matter with me?' I thought. 'Am I becoming a sex maniac?' "

"Well, doesn't Donna treat you all right?" his friend asked.

"Yeah, Donna's okay," Jim retorted. "But, well, she works hard, is a good mother, but we don't have anything going."

"What the hell does that mean?" his friend questioned.

"There's no spark; even sex has become routine. She and I have talked about it ... twenty years is a long time with one woman."

"Hey, Donna's a good-looking gal," his friend countered. "Not potty like half the gals in our neighborhood."

"True ... but it's not exciting. I even bought *The Joy of Sex,* but she's not interested.

"You know, old George wasn't dead three days when I started hustling Sally, his secretary. Sally, she is so sexy! She's young, and exciting, a real beauty. ... Isn't that crazy?"

Jim's symptoms are many—fears, loneliness, and changing life-forces that affect all his anchors. Let's look at some of these anchors or areas of change.

One area of change in male metapause is a growing dissatisfaction with our work. Once we were anointed to go far. We pinned our hopes on the company, only to have the hopes give way to mid-life mumblings around the water cooler: "I'm in a rut." The nine-to-five scene is no longer appealing. With guys in the company collapsing at their desks, and a few sixty-year-old senior partners keeping us in our places we wonder what we're doing. We feel more like "cogs in a machine." Progress, so what! Higher sales, longer forecasts, so what!

Now, it's our subordinates who bring up new ideas, and we react in two unusual ways: first, we try to recall the last time we came up with a new idea, and second, we get that sinking feeling in our stomachs as we realize that the implementation of the idea would make a ten-hour day a twelve-hour one, just when we feel a need for rest or diversion.

Along with the tired feeling in staff meetings at work, other physical changes affect us. After a day long meeting, we return home and fall asleep in the easy chair in front of the TV. We look into the mirror while shaving, and find we've changed, our faces are falling. We have longer hair, which no longer covers the bald spot. We do sit-ups every morning, play golf or jog, but no matter what we do, the weight continues to increase. This is all a part of The Gray Itch.

We also have some questions about our continued athletic prowess, another shattered mirror of who we are. Taking the ski chair lift becomes the challenge; and skiing down the hill, a rosary of our Blue Cross numbers. We want more than ever to relate to the opposite sex, but after we hug someone we must back up beyond arm's length to see who it is. We keep our glasses on when we go to bed, only to have the damn glasses fog up!

We find that names and numbers are slow to emerge from our memory. We tend to forget where a client lives or what his favorite drink is. We feel a little like the college professor who said to his class, "I shall now illustrate what I have in mind," and then proceeded to erase the blackboard. In summary, we spent the first forty years having our minds and bodies prove who we are, and the next forty years will be spent checking it out to see if it's still there.

Another area where the changing "Who am I?" of The Gray Itch exists is in bed. Some forty-year-old syndrome men wonder what will happen to their performance record every time they go to bed. Others screw themselves to death. Other metapausal types get panicky when they get that early-evening look from their wives. Still others on business trips pick up some young chick, only to wonder why. Many fantasize about having affairs. Some have them, only to conclude that they really just wanted to see if they could have one.

We evaluated our marriages in the past through sexual encounters. As encounters become fewer and fewer, and performances less predictable, we begin to disagree with the University of Wisconsin newspaper slogan that said that those who lay together, stay together.

Family life is changing, too. Our overriding purpose at an

earlier time now seems to be a drag. Many feel their family relationships are but business enterprises: braces, cars, prom dresses, plumbing bills, aspirin, 10½ percent interest payments and, of course, college, the place everybody goes.

We find that the business enterprise at home isn't enough. We need closeness, care, intimacy.

Breakfast becomes a serial process with each member of the household eating at fifteen-minute feeding intervals before splitting in six different directions.

The first five minutes in the door at night are the most traumatic of the day. Common remarks are: "The washer is broken," or "The lawn is dying," or "I broke my front tooth today, Dad," or "Get ready, remember we're going over to the Lawrences' for dinner."

Like the encounter at the front door, the dinner table is often a chorus of grunts and moans that nothing important ever happens. The scale of cost-and-effort in the enterprise and the members' lack of expressed satisfaction or involvement in each other are out of whack. We begin to dare ask whether the business at home seems all too much like the business at work. We wonder, "What am I? A businessman? A father? A person? Where's the 'me' in all this?" We scratch ourselves, but The Gray Itch persists.

If some of this family life seems familiar to you, you may have some symptoms of the forty-year-old syndrome. Stranded in an outmoded set of roles, we become stranded in ourselves.

Another area of the metapausal syndrome relates to our wives. Remember the Doris Day of the Class of '50? Has she become just another client or associate in the family business enterprise? Like us, she is busy. She is involved in more guilds than a Florentine artist. Her family sees much less of her, as she puts 30,000 miles a year on the family car. And she tops off your week by telling you she is going to enroll in the local university for a few courses.

We have trouble remembering anything really personal between our wives and ourselves—a conversation, a touch. Some research indicates that personal communication between couples married fifteen years or more is about seventeen minutes a week. Think of it! Seventeen minutes a week! Try to think of four personal—not business—concerns that you and your wife have expressed to each other in the last two weeks. You can think of only one? Well, you're not alone. We seldom talk to each other about personal things without a constant barrage of interruptions by the junior partners.

Sometimes we are aware of this lack of communication, so we take the wife out to dinner. We hope we don't look like those other forty-year-old couples sitting in a restaurant or bar, looking off into space like the figures in a Degas painting. We simply have little to say at these "Annual Dinner Meetings," for we each manage a different part of the enterprise.

Ah, yes, the kids—our pride and joy, chips off the old block, direct reflections of us. Are they still mirrors of who we are? Their lives are so involved in their own activities they seem but numbers in the family bank account—college trust. When the family conversation does take place, it generally gets heated and ends when the kids say, "That's your opinion, Dad," or, "Sure, Dad. Sure, Dad." Out of frustration, we give the kids the old "when-I-was-your-age" bit or other famous generation-gap tune-outs. As the family confusion increases and the self-doubt grows in us, the self-image fogs. We wonder if we are bus driver, mediator, treasurer, chairman of the board, or office boy for the enterprise.

And our parents can be a problem, too. At a time when they need us more, we help them—but sometimes feel caught between generations.

One further problem in metapause is the fact that the house and community or "the place" we live really doesn't mean much anymore. After years of Boy Scouts, paper drives, school board meetings, Gray Y, ecology hikes, and membership on the stop-sign committee (you know, the one you were instrumental in having placed at Oak Street), you've had it. And the house itself not only costs a lot every month, but every time we turn around, it needs painting, weeding, or a new faucet. Worn out like the faucet washers, we feel the pressure that lessens the pride we once had in "my house." With it goes yet another point establishing who we are.

Coupled with the incessant interest on the part of your wife in moving to Upper Elm Street, where interest rates are out of sight, is enough for many men to turn left at Oak Street. Beyond the civic duties and the house, the neighborhood is changing. Old Ralph got transferred; your regular foursome is but a memory. There are no more Christmas carolers, and the new next-door neighbors have small children and a big dog that prefers your lawn—which took fifteen years to grow—to his own.

As the family money machine, do you now find you're looking to buy more things—for yourself? It's a common symptom of the Gray Itch, as telltale as is a sore throat. Maybe a sportscar, new golf clubs, a Playboy Club membership, larger sportscoats in brighter colors, or a new, twenty-five-dollar hairstyle? Many of us now feel it's time we spent something on ourselves; a Porsche or a Jaguar is the least we owe ourselves. We may end up like old George, slumped over our desks, so why not live a little? And one allowable way to live in our materialistic society is to "buy it up" a little.

At 46, you may feel that you've been fired from all of your jobs. In the subway, on that freeway drive home, even during an occasional family dinner, does loneliness and mild depression often come over you without warning? This loneliness can lead to self-doubt or at least insecurity, as the popular song relates: "I'm sad to be alone. I hope I make it through the night." Have you made a telephone call home, said "Hi," only to have one of your offspring on the other end say, "Who is this?"

If these areas of male metapause give you a certain itch, you've got it, The Gray Itch! You may be suffering from a mild or severe case, the conditions caused by changes in how we have defined ourselves that insidiously creep up on us as we reach mid-life.

Chapter 3

MY I.D. IS SLIPPING

The male metapause syndrome is a navigational system gone haywire, an old radio we need to hit to get our favorite station. It's the disorientation we get when we walk to our car, only to find it's parked on the other side of the lot. Like a blind man, the middle-aged man feels his way in mid-life, listening to the sound of his stick as he approaches a curb—listening for a new stage of life.

Past mirrors of identity or "Who am I?" the wife, the kids, the job, sexual and physical self are changing. Daddy and vice-president roles have been played out, and become as useful in defining who you are as an appendix or an earlobe. These mirrors just don't fit us anymore. Metapause is a time when roles and identities are caught in between, This in-between time of The Gray Itch is called an identity crisis by psychologists, a time when "my I.D. is slipping."

Understanding our tentativeness, confusion, or even crisis, our feeling of being the middle scoop in a three-decker cone can be infinitely easier if we look at how identity develops throughout life stages. One aerospace engineer put it this way:

If I had known at 25 what I know now at 50 ... for example, generally what the road ahead would be like, its expectations of me and me of it, I would have been much more intelligent about me, less critical, less blaming of others, less dreaming and wanting. More a man and less a boy.

We will, then, speed up the camera of life and, like an old Keystone Cop comedy, show how our identity develops through life stages and the roles they lead us to play as we move down the road. Again, our progress in understanding ourselves seems to begin with metathoughts, thoughts of our own life span: "If I only had it to do over again." "You only go around once." "Is this the summer or the fall of my life?" "I wonder if I can last until the kids graduate." "Ten more years and I can get out of this company."

Comparing Life Cycles

To get the idea of how life stages affect who we are, let's contrast the life cycle of Joe, an aboriginal Indian of Tasmania, to that of our own.

In Joe's society, there *isn't* a middle life. Life expectancy is thirty years. The primitive moves rapidly from child-producing age to death. We can see that Joe's life is largely determined by its span. Our life expectancy is seventy-two years plus, resulting from a unique yet perplexing gift given us by an exceptionally advanced society.

Because Joe's life cycle is shortened, child rearing also takes less time than in our culture. At nine, his son begins the rites of passage and his teeth are knocked out, as within the Arunta culture. At fourteen, he's circumcised and he becomes a man. To Joe, raising children doesn't seem to be such a big deal. A long and doting preoccupation is only common among industrialized Western humanity. Statements like "But think of the children, dear," or "We must put more money away for Larry's tuition," could hardly become the national anthem in Tasmania.

Further contrast shows that Joe's sons wish to be like him; Joe doesn't long to be like his sons. He doesn't wear their necklaces; they will wear his someday. Unlike American society, where a twenty-year-old feels disgust because he's at the pinnacle of life and his father is downhill, Joe's sons are looking forward to being older.

At twenty-five, toward the end of his life, Joe goes through rites of passage again. He becomes a spiritual leader. Contrast that with old Harry at Oak Street. Joe, an elder, a family priest, becomes part of the most respected generation. But when Harry says, "That's the way it was in the old days," the young people around the pool look at him as if he's had too much vodka and grapefruit juice. Projecting themselves into a future of serial marriages, extrasensory communication, Venus vacations, and a hundred-year life cycle, Harry's kids think, "What's an old man know, anyway?" This statement in Joe's culture would get any fifteen-year-old beaten with sticks and banished—not to his room with his stereo, motorcycle posters, fish tank, and girl friend, but out of the tribe and beyond tradition.

Joe's initiation as an elder, leader, and wise man of the tribe makes his last years very meaningful to him. He doesn't have any trepidation about death, whereas death is the American middle-aged male's special preoccupation. Joe's already a member of the club as a living elder.

As a special reward, Joe gets the pick of most of the young women as he ages. Joe knows who he is sexually. He has an early and continual sexual experience. Sexual prowess isn't much of a preoccupation in Joe's case. In the Western male cycle, we grow pubic hair nearly ten years before we sanction its exposure to the opposite sex. Here, education, religion, and fighting our wars all delay sexual gratification. In the very short period from age twenty to thirty, the tradition of the Western world holds the male should enjoy himself sexually. After that time, it's a declining market, or so he is told.

Joe's culture hasn't changed in a thousand years. As an elder, he transmits to the young the tribe's traditions. Contrast Joe with Harry, the middle-aged American suffering from future shock, living in a house with members of another, younger generation who speak in a strange tongue, dress and act as if they were from a country other than the one they grew up in. Because life is unchanging, decisions and directions for Joe are predicated primarily on the past. Old Harry can hardly pay for his new car before it falls apart. Joe deals in absolutes; Harry can't. In American industry, any reference stated in the past tense causes eyebrows to raise around the board table. "Old Harry must be slowing down," they whisper at the end of the table. "A retirement village for him—a Leisure World." And, like so many others, old Harry becomes an industrial castoff.

But alas, even Joe doesn't have it all together. All is not young girls and wise ceremonials. Occasionally his identity slips when one of his younger women is attracted to a young warrior, or one of his sons rivals him. The latter is uncommon, however, since Joe will die about the time his son becomes old enough to be a power in the family. No two men are under the same roof, and Joe knows it. Contrast this with families in this country today, where a grandfather in full health, a middle-aged father, and a twenty-five-year-old son all live under the same roof.

Life Stages

When we look further at the Western male's life stages, three points must be considered briefly. First, most of us are constantly working out conflicts in whatever stage we happen to be. The good news is that this struggle is expected and normal in healthy individuals. The bad news is that it's a lifetime process and we never seem to quite finish the struggle.

The linking of our life stages becomes the second point. One stage is mostly resolved before moving to the next one. However, when a stage remains largely *un*resolved, we tend to carry the residue of conflict into the next stage. An example is the perennial teenager.

Now let's look at how stages in our life cycle have molded who we are at metacenter, and what we expect from the stages yet to come:

We'll follow the life-stage development model fashioned by Erik H. Erikson, whose clinical work and writing have become the standard in this area. Erikson has not related his developmental stages directly to middle-aged men, so, for the sake of brevity and necessary interpretation, what follows only partially refers to his theory.[1]

Stage 1: Trust versus Mistrust

Early in our lives we develop a feeling of trust and mistrust. Trust is an important issue as we move toward independence, and toward intimacy in later stages. To be able to trust our own feelings is to be able to interact as a responsible person without undue suspicion of others or ourselves.

Stage 2: Autonony versus Shame and Doubt

As we grow, trust becomes autonomy. "Some develop a will or wish to be on their own, to assume a sense of autonomy, to stand on their own two feet—an important issue in personal identity," Erikson points out.[2]

In these early stages trust and autonomy are exceedingly important reflections of who we will be in middle-age.

Stage 3: Initiation versus Guilt

In childhood we learn to initiate or withdraw through guilt. We walk away from our mothers, only to return; we walk to the edge of the surf, only to return quickly to our parents as the wave reaches us. We initiate on our own, we separate ourselves, we discover new things, we discover risk—an important ingredient for the middle-aged man's development.

Stage 4: Industry versus Inferiority

Continuing our interpretation and applying it to middle-aged men, we are now well into our search for "Who am I?" and enter the stage where payoff revolves around how industrious we are—from model airplanes to a good report card, from working on a ham radio to being a basketball star. Industry results in products that are appreciated by both friends and parents. We get complimented often: "Great airplane, Jerry." "That was a fine basketball game you played today, Joe." These are strokes for our future productivity. If we don't succeed, we try and try again. We begin to become that which we produce. Many men find their jobs to be who they are, part of what Karl Marx called "the craft idiocy."

Stage 5: Identity versus Role Confusion
Now we enter adolescence, that very perplexing and painful period in our life cycle. Equipped with the results of previous development such as trust, autonomy, initiation, and industry, youth is propelled into adolescence. Adolescents become the guerrilla army against the adult world, defining themselves through strange talk and dress. Spirited by wearing fatigues, having a van, strumming a guitar, and speaking a few irrational grunts, this time of moratorium allows those in their teens the last vestiges of youth. Emerging from this stage takes several years. "A boundary seems to exist between the individual and the adult world for many years," Douglas Kimmell observes.[3]

Stage 6: Intimacy versus Isolation
Although sexual intimacy may have begun to develop during our teens at a drive-in, a well-developed and intimate relationship may not develop until late into the thirties for many. For some it never occurs. Care for other persons develops during this stage. This special sense of caring can develop only if there is a real appreciation for self. Erikson has said:

Sexual intimacy is only part of what I have in mind, for it is obvious that sexual intimacy does often precede the capacity to develop a true and mutual psycho-social intimacy with another person. The intimate friendship, erotic encounters are joint inspiration. The youth who is not sure of his identity shies away from interpersonal intimacy and throws himself into acts of intimacy which are promiscuous, without true fusion or self-abandon.[4]

Further interpretation of Erikson indicates all of these previous stages are important to the ultimate development of intimacy—the ability to share, to care, and to dare. Roger Gould of U.C.L.A. points out: "Throughout the years of adulthood, there is an ever-increasing need to win permission from oneself to continue developing."[5]
Unfortunately, during this time another cycle of life, the

work cycle, intervenes and vies with developing intimacy. Being your own man and caring for others are often sublimated to our work ethic. As males, our attention is turned toward a career, or "making it." Acts of caring are intentionally forced out of the race. The "hardheaded" dominates the "sensitive" and the "affectionate."

Vacillating as he does in his late twenties and early thirties between the needs for industry and intimacy, the male begins to question where previous stages have taken him. Sometime between the ages of thirty-five and fifty-five, his life stages confuse him. He sits behind his desk fourteen hours a day on the one hand, yet dreams of closeness on the other. He questions his industry stage. "I'm tired of work" becomes "I need an affair." Amid The Gray Itch identity loss or confusion, the middle-aged man reaches yet another stage.

Stage 7: Generativity versus Stagnation

Here the middle-aged man begins to think about generativity, which represents producing something that will outlive him (not just making a quota). In this stage, the "early industry stage" takes a back seat to his driving interest in deeper relationships with others and his needs for fulfillment. One-night stands are no longer adequate, if they ever were. Affection returns to him—even for his competition—and boredom, lack of goals, obsolescence, and overspecialization lead him to say, "Is that all there is?" We want more control over our work. We desire to teach others what we do, to become mentors for younger colleagues. Adding to our generativity, we want something that will outlive us, something more than a gold watch at retirement.

"Is that all there is?," a mid-life slogan of stagnation, forces middle-aged men to seek beyond their boredom and confusion for reaffirmation. Making it into generativity and beyond, the middle-aged man struggles to win at a point of crisis in the seventh stage. Great men such as Freud, Jung, O'Neill, Frank Lloyd Wright, Goya, and Gandhi are examples of some who did it.

Not making it means stagnation—last week's *TV Guide,* last

summer's fruit punch, last night's failure in bed. Stagnation is a black mask placed over the head on the long line of those to be executed, hanged by the neck until dead by lack of understanding of life stages. Take Sam, for example: "I feel like I'm gradually disintegrating. I've learned to shuffle. I walk like a Cook County Hospital inmate. I can pick up my feet when I walk, but I don't want to. Picking up your feet all these years takes a lot out of a guy."

In the late forties and early fifties, a mellowing out of feelings and relationships seems to occur. We desire to become human once again; jobs fall into perspective. Some metapausal men become eager for human experience. Sharing of joys, sorrows, and confusion doesn't represent weakness to them as it once did.

Instead of searching for the glitter and power of tomorrow, deep feelings or doing something for someone else defines the value of being.

Robert C. Peck, a noted researcher, has observed that a sense of openness develops as a part of generativity. Being open to life's flexibility, being able to change, to hang loose. To ride and tame future shock; not to go back to the good old days, but ahead as well; not just to go toward old friends but to form new acquaintances.[6]

We might further interpret generativity as a time of putting the physical self aside; there don't seem to be that many George Blandas around.

Stage 8: Ego Integrity versus Despair

Each stage in this lifelong process of "Who am I?" relates to Ego Integration versus Despair. Now we reach the last stage as developed by Erikson:

Only in him who in some way has taken care of things and people and who has adapted himself to the triumphs and disappointments inherent in being, the originating of others or in the generating of products and ideas, only in him may gradually reap the fruit of the seven stages.[7]

Here we get a feeling like paying off the mortgage, or "when we become, finally, our own men," as Dan Levinson of Yale has called it.

Some of the markings of integration are companionship and a sense of closeness. Here we find the middle-aged (or older) man integrating his work into his life, not his life into his work. Unlike in the time and stage when he stood before his father holding the model airplane, saying, "I did it, I did it," the middle-aged man looks at his product as only a single extension of his expanded "Who am I?"—and probably not the most important one at that.

Here in the integrated personality, "If I only had it to do over again" is but a cry of despair and a statement of little meaning. In this stage, amid the scar tissue of disappointment, emerges the gift of meaning.

It becomes clear as we look at the stages of trust, autonomy, industry, intimacy, generativity, and integrity, that the metapausal man is truly a product of his life cycle.

Certain questions about who he is follow naturally with each adult developmental stage. Shakespeare recognized that in these familiar lines from *As You Like It:*

All the world's a stage and all the men and women merely players. They have their exits and their entrances, and one man in his time plays many parts. His acts being seven ages.

At first, the infant, mewling and puking in his nurse's arms, then the whining schoolboy with his satchel and shining morning face, creeping like a snail, unwillingly to school. And then the lover, sighing like a furnace with a woeful ballad made to his mistress' eyebrow. Then a soldier, full of strange oaths and bearded like the pard, jealous in honor, sudden and quick in quarrel, seeking the bubble reputation even in the cannon's mouth. And then the justice, in fair round belly with good capon lin'd, with eyes severe and beard of formal cut, full of wise saws and modern instances; and so he plays his part.

The sixth stage shifts into the lean and slipper'd pantaloon, with spectacles on nose and pouch on side; his youthful hose, well sav'd, a world too wide for his shrunk shank, and his big manly voice, turning again toward childish treble, pipes and whistles in his sound. Last scene of all, that ends this strange eventful history, is second childishness and mere oblivion, sans teeth, sans eyes, sans taste, sans everything.

Roles We Play

Along with the mid-life confusion described earlier, the roles that we have been taught, conditioned for and expected to play plague us. These roles—some fixed, some obsolete—are played over and over again until who we are becomes a worn record on the turntable. Playing the tunes of the 1950s, we listen to these roles we wished to be—father, husband, vice-president.

Roles that we acted out in the past wrap us in tinsel, protecting the changing person inside from being discovered. As we enter into generativity, we feel changes are needed and we begin to take fewer curtain calls for the roles we played in the past.

We feel much like the fellow who said: "At Harry's champagne Christmas party, I acted badly. As a respected vice-president of Amalgamated, and Sally's husband, I tried to break out of the old roles and get a special pre-Christmas present from a redhead with half a Santa's outfit on."

A quiet desperation and confusion ensues. Sometimes even an urgency plagues us. A sense of role entrapment reminds us of a previous time when we played an expected role. Remember "U.S. 25621814, Corporal, Second Regiment." Remember getting up early at five o'clock to face another long day of playing roles that weren't you—watching the same re-ups playing poker, looking straight ahead in the latrine, marching in a column of ducks. All were a part of your role as Corporal, U.S. Army.

While your roles were fixed and understood, didn't you have trouble being you? Now, in mid-life, you feel somewhat the same. Only today "your ass" belongs to you . . . or does it? Over the years, have you traded one set of numbers for doing a number as vice-president of Amalgamated . . . or as a family banker . . . or as a respected member of the community? Have you merely traded your dogtags for another set?

By mid-life, you thought you would have become somebody, somebody unique . . . you. If you haven't made it (like many of us other corporals), you feel like a number much of the time. Maybe you're still 256215814. And now you want out of the outfit. As a person, you don't seem to count very much. Maybe that's it—maybe you're not a person, you're a set of roles.

We ask where and when did the confusion start, what caused it? Did I get it in the Army, or did I get it when I turned forty? Why do I speed from New York to Connecticut, downtown to the lake or L.A., to the Valley metathinking about "me."

We hear ourselves acting out roles we no longer appreciate or get satisfaction from. At work we say, "I've got the door, J.B.," or at home, "I'll decide when we buy a new car," or, "As long as you're my son, you will." Hearing the echo of our out-of-date roles indicates something is happening to us and others around us. Today our bed partners want to be more like us. Today, we're not the chairman but the chairperson. We're no longer the only provider, we have a joint income. We're not even the final word. Practicing well-fixed roles that we have learned on the one hand and sharing these roles on the other often causes the middle-aged man double vision.

Today, your inner self shouts metathoughts: "I'm more than somebody's father, more than a company man! I've been playacting, not really being me. I've suppressed myself because of responsibilities I had for my family, the society, and others." Again, Gould adds to our interpretation:

Each role in life can lead to two opposite results in the change process. A role can be an opportunity to come to a more comprehensive understanding of oneself in action, or a role can become a simplified definition of a self that does not do justice to the whole, complex human being.[8]

Identity is learned and played out through role statements within a particular pattern of life staging. Within this context, we are now ready to look at the influence of changes within our "Who am I?"

To understand our identity crisis, we must look at other players on our team—our wives, our children, our jobs, our physical and sexual selves. It seems that the key to a traumatic male metapause syndrome relates to the changes in these first-team members as well as in ourselves. In subsequent chapters we'll examine each of these roles and players and try to analyze how our identities become confused and distended in middle age—remembering that identity is never a final achievement, as Erikson has said. "It's anything but static and unchanging"; it's a continuous search for "me."

Part II
LET ME OUT
OF HERE!

Chapter 4

VICE-PRESIDENT WHO?

Turning right or left on Oak Street each morning presents an important dilemma. Left means a supposed freedom, excitement, stimulation. Right means going to work.

Remember the days when your electric garage door was the first one up in the morning and your office lights were the last off at night? Remember how proud you were when Amalgamated got that big contract? *You* were the one responsible for beating out the competition at old Consolidated. You were selected as the youngest vice-president to present a new product line at the annual meeting. And don't forget that twelfth-floor office with the big mahogany desk covered with exciting forecasts, airline tickets, buck slips, locks on *all* the drawers, and the telephone console with the strange buttons? You didn't even have to go down the hall to the john, you had your own. Those were the days! The sky was the limit!

What happened? Why do you now, in middle age, question whether to go to work or to turn left on Oak Street?

Instead of skip-stopping the stop sign at Oak Street and charging off to work as you did in the old days, you sit behind the crosswalk, arms over the top of the steering wheel, daydreaming. "I'm not going in today," you mumble. "I'm going fishin' or to the beach." Your daydreaming continues into that second cup of coffee during the break, the three-hour lunch on Friday, or the early-hour martinis before going home.

You are in a job crisis, a significant part of male metapause and one which Dero Saunders says will face most forty- to fifty-year-old executives in medium-sized to large U.S. corporations today. He called it "an executive menopause." This middle-aged job crisis is what *Time* magazine called "The Second Act in American Life." [1]

This crisis is typical of the metapausal man, representing more than half of the forty-seven million middle-aged workers in America. As one counselor reports about a client:

The first interview I had with a man suffering from this condition made an indelible impression on me. He was 42 years old, good-looking, had money and recognition. He was the leading attorney in the community and his name was well-known to me. He just came in and asked that I get him a job in another field. I have talked to dozens of attorneys, teachers, ministers and managers—all faced with this same occupational dilemma—since that first interview. [2]

Like many middle-aged men in counseling, you now have trouble getting up for the big contracts. Once you negotiated and enjoyed the infighting, the struggle, the competition, didn't you? What happened?

After years of the dollar squeeze, continuous changes in product line, new quotas, territories, and competitors, you feel the whole thing is a drag.

In some ways, it seems to be you, it's not the job alone. Witness the following metathoughts: "I'm not with it anymore." "I feel trapped." "I'm scared." "For the first time, I seem to feel I'm slipping at work." "With the new sales quotas, I feel like I must start over every year."

Work Identity

The middle-aged man feels a sense of entrapment, caused by fears of routine, overspecialization, obsolescence, lack of goals, competition, or a career clock that is out of whack. Before we explore these elements, it's important to understand how deeply entwined each middle-aged man is with his work roles.

According to Cyril Sofer, work roles contribute to personal identity.[3] They provide an opportunity to define oneself to others, enter into a stable set of relations with colleagues or clients, and explain one's place in the world. To a large degree, the American male *is* his work. He "lives to work" instead of "works to live." It is estimated that men identify upwards of 60 to 80 percent of "who they are" through work relationships.

Occupational success and satisfaction "reaffirms the individual's sense of identity" and provides "social recognition" for that identity, according to Douglas C. Kimmel.[4] Kenneth Soddy feels that an occupation is perhaps a man's "major emotional satisfaction." [5]

To many, this overidentification with work may seem exaggerated. A couple of exercises may bring the point home. First, spend some time talking with a stranger and try not to mention what you do. The person with whom you're speaking will continually probe to find out what your work is. You will find it difficult not to talk of your work in attempting to describe who you are.

Now, bring to mind the first question you were asked at a recent cocktail party or dinner. From this one simple question, "What do you do?," a whole series of roles and identifying characteristics are established. The person now knows something about your education, something about where you live, how much money you make, and what your job responsibility happens to be. Unfortunately, he knows little about you as a person.

Conditioning to commingle the American male's self-concept with his work starts at a very young age. From kindergarten, we can recall "being" a fireman, a policeman, or a pilot. Early in high school, people would prejudge us by asking, "What does your father do?" From our first job of mowing the neighbor's lawn to later owning our own appliance store, work has given us rewards: money, wheels, and the right to have Susie. This conditioning toward being industrious eventually forms itself into an overriding desire for us "to have a good job someday." A clear translation is, "I want to be a successful person."

This same conditioning leads to a schedule for success in a career. Since careers are age-graded, certain positions are desired by men of certain ages.

One study reported that occupational aspirations change around age thirty-five. At this age, emphasis shifts from measuring success in terms of achievement to measuring it in terms of economic security.[6]

C. Sofer feels "Work provides the individual with a situation where he is both expected and accepted," and sustains a man's place in his social network.[7]

As mentioned earlier, the American male is his work, and Len, an insurance salesman and a client in group counseling, said:

I have a hard time when someone criticizes my work. I'm a real expert in my field. When someone criticizes me, I get childish about it. I sulk. Maybe I'm too close to my work, maybe a vacation would help. But where would I go? I can't afford it, and I never developed any hobbies. I guess ... I guess I feel trapped by my work, and yet what else am I?

If an inseparable tie between the American male and his work exists, what happens in mid-life when the wind is taken out of our sails at work?

"I Feel Trapped"

Several things occur that change the way we look at our work in mid-life and add to our Gray Itch.

The formal definition of "entrapment" has several properties: being snared, allowing one to go through while catching another, to draw into contradiction. Each has special relevance to the fifty-year-old and his work.

Being snared or caught "in the system" represents the first definition of entrapment, which develops out of feelings of routine, obsolescence, and overspecialization. While he is part of the first or second generation (in large numbers), to enjoy a thirty- or forty-year career, the technology demands ever newer models with a new set of competencies required each decade.

The second definition of entrapment means allowing one to pass through while catching the other. This form of entrapment is represented by competition, mobility, and lack of goals. Of those qualified to be president of the company, only one gets the nod or the big contract. When poor old Sam is transferred from one coast to the other, that's just the way it goes.

According to studies by the U.S. Department of Labor, movement up the occupational ladder is largely completed by around age thirty-five, and chances are that those who haven't achieved their career goals by the forties or fifties will never do it and may actually slip down the career ladder.[8]

A counselor of middle-aged men reacted to this problem when he said:

Despite all the emphasis on executive development, a guy over 45 has a hell of a time getting a job; and even at 45, he doesn't have the freedom to move anymore. At 45, you're caught in a cultural trap.[9]

The third definition of entrapment means drawing one into contradiction. The contradiction lies in our time and place and our commitment to our work. Many a middle-aged man is unable to move ahead in the company but finds retirement will barely pay the bills; entrapment means looking back and finding it's too late to start again, and looking forward to retirement and finding it's too far away.

Especially chafing to the middle-rank executive of forty or forty-five is the fact that *his* boss is taking his own sweet time in retiring. When the boss gets to be fifty-five or sixty, he explains: "I meant to retire at fifty-five but changed my mind. I have standing here, I'm looked up to, and I'm recognized as a member of the team. I don't want to lose that." His forty-five-year-old subordinate sees him letting down, lacking the drive and technical equipment. His reaction is, "What's wrong with that guy? He's got money, he could go fishing or do anything he likes. Why doesn't he leave?"

Many seem to need greater control of their work. R.

Blauner's review of work satisfaction underlies the extent to which opportunities for autonomy have been found to affect men's assessments of satisfaction at work.[10]

Instead of looking for new opportunities, the middle-aged man looks for more care, feeding, and protection by the company. Herein lies the contradiction. On the one hand, he wishes to separate himself a little more from his job. Being just "vice-president who" and being less of his own man no longer appeals to him. However, fear of not getting ahead causes him to take a stronger grip on the trapeze and to let go of his autonomy, an important quality of identifying who he is in the world.

This is a downward spiral. For many less able to separate themselves from their work or grab a greater sense of autonomy from it, work satisfaction decreases and greater feelings of entrapment ensue. Those who "take a larger grip on the company" often feel that they are more disposable and have "white knuckles" until retirement.

Several clues to this feeling of entrapment and the elements that cause it, then, are found in work mobility, obsolescence, specialization, competition, goal orientation, and routine.

"Hey, I Want to Settle Down"

Ironically, one of the major areas of entrapment comes from moving around. The middle-aged man relates to a piece of turf that is his—107 Elm Street, Jefferson High, or his desk. He's tired of I.B.M.—"I've Been Moved." After years of pulling up stakes for this or that promotion, the panic of entrapment comes over him when the boss calls him into the office and talks about "that fantastic opportunity in Seattle." The man who's run the shop out in Podunk for twenty years has developed deep roots. He doesn't want to move.

Referring to job mobility, the U.S. Department of Labor cites evidence that some mobile middle-aged workers trade off gains in some job characteristics, such as earnings, for losses in others, namely satisfaction. It also cites rates of mobility between major occupation groups of middle-aged men as between 17 and 25 percent with professionals and technicians among the least mobile and sales workers among the most mobile.[11] Statements of middle-aged men in one study regarding job mobility included: "One learns never to turn down promotions because one would be labeled unambitious."[12]

Entrapment feelings about job mobility run counter to feelings of settling in. Remember Willie Lohman, the protagonist of Arthur Miller's *Death of a Salesman,* when he said: "I tell you why, Howard. Speaking frankly, and just between the two of us, y'know—I'm just a little tired."

How much do you feel like Willie—afraid to join the country club for fear of losing your nonrefundable membership fee? How about that mountain cabin that you always wanted for your older years—should you build it in California or on the coast of Maine? Does your baseball-playing son need to look in the yearbook to find out what his school colors are? Do you always mark "visitor" at church?

At first, moving to Connecticut, Palo Alto, and Denver were exciting. But years of change-of-address cards and coast-to-coast dittoed Christmas letters make one say, "What's the use—I'll just coast in."

Job mobility upsets our need for a place. And loneliness and separation are accompanying experiences. Remember as a kid the first time you went to camp? Remember when you left for college or for the war?

We require a territory to define who we are. Like nearly all animals, from the African cob, who sits on his mound, to the hippo, who at certain times of the year draws a circle of dung around his place with his belly, we all need a territory. This territorial imperative is also true of man, even if it's only Archie Bunker's chair. Ever watch the territoriality of those who come to a staff meeting? They always sit in the same place, don't they?

Job mobility insidiously breaks down our definition of self and territory in mid-life. During the twenties and thirties the company man forfeits much of his turf for opportunity. The corporate man's easy chair has spent at least two of the last twenty years in a moving van.

If we have moved often, we don't seem interested in becoming involved in our new community. No more stop-sign committees for us. We become tentative, afraid to commit ourselves, fearful of that inevitable call from the boss: "Jim, you'll love Baltimore." Instead, we see how many potted plants we can get into the moving van, and we coordinate the harvest of the vegetable garden with the presentation of the annual report.

So, one day, we get our backs up and say, "The hell with Baltimore. I'm staying here." We hear the boss on the other end of the line say, "Okay, Jim, it's up to you." And we know very well that, after twenty-five years of valuable service, a special notation is being made in our personnel files: "Somewhat unwilling to move."

Unlike the Gypsies, who take their community and friends with them, the family that moves to Baltimore must develop an entirely new group of interpersonal relationships at work and in the neighborhood. The feeling of closeness and togetherness in a community is an impossible dream for many a corporate executive, and becomes a direct cause of loneliness for him in mid-life.

Every person needs personal stability and social continuity. In mid-life, we may need it more than most. Is it any wonder we feel uncertain, tentative about our work, tired of being a short-timer?

Note some of these conditions in George, a California aerospace engineer with a master's degree, who spent the last ten years with six different companies, and who, a couple of years ago, found himself without a job:

I began to question myself in a lot of ways—my skills, my education, my value as a person. Worst of all, I stopped caring if I ever found a new job. I was tired of moving from one company to another—I felt like my son's hamster on its treadmill, running and running but never getting anywhere. Besides, a new job might mean moving to another area, and I just couldn't go through that again.

"I Feel Like a Retread"

Other culprits of our entrapment within our work today are obsolescence and overspecialization. Feelings of insecurity result when a middle-aged man sees his younger colleagues promoted faster than he into positions of status traditionally reserved for the middle generation. Again, Soddy feels this threat to the self-image is responsible for the decline in efficiency, increase in rigidity, and inability to compete characteristic of many middle-aged workers.[13]

How many times have we sat in a staff meeting with a tight feeling in our stomach, feeling outdated, wondering what's wrong with us, as in Tim's case:

I really am loyal to the company. But it's funny, at staff meetings I seem to just sit there, the younger attorneys seem to monopolize the entire meeting. Every time I want to say something, they beat me to the punch. I just don't seem to be aggressive anymore. I seem to sit by and listen to them, or sometimes even drop out altogether and think about my secretary's legs or going to Tahiti.

And when I try to get into the conversation, it's amazing how resentment comes out of me toward those young bastards in the fancy suits and the shiny new degrees, spitting out precedents left and right, precedents I've never heard of.

What's wrong with me? They help the partnership as well as I do, they're good attorneys. Do I resent them just because they're younger? I guess I resent being pushed around by these young people. Yet, they don't seem to be basically more capable than I am. Deep down in my heart, maybe I'm afraid. I'm afraid of not getting my senior partner's slot, and maybe I'm afraid of becoming obsolete.

This feeling is repeated hundreds of times in all professions, by middle-aged men every day. We are men who have spent countless seventy-hour weeks, and then one day a metathought comes to mind: "I'm a throw-away, a nondeposit."

Our technology is an insatiable glutton. It receives its nutrition from the energy and knowledge of all of us. When our special energy and knowledge becomes tough and gristly, the technology spits us out. While it is busily chewing up fourth-generation computer personnel, why should it be stuck with a menu of middle-aged, second-generation personnel? Technology's use of us is bad enough, but even worse is *our* discovery that we might be out of date.

"I Know More and More about Less and Less"

Overspecialization leads to yet another form of entrapment for the middle-aged man. You've become a specialist over the years, narrowing your depth and developing your expertise. Learning more and more about less and less, being the man in the know.

One group-counseling experience comes to mind about two aerospace engineers who had specialized in propeller-driven landing gear assemblies, who suddenly found themselves working in a corporation that did nothing but rocketry.

Entrapped in our own work specialties, we sit at staff meetings and have trouble understanding the other specialists. Not unlike a U.N. meeting, or lunch at a university faculty club, we all speak different languages—those of our specialties. Technology keeps chewing up advanced knowledge at a faster and faster rate, and acres and acres of previously qualified personnel become the fields of stalks after last year's harvest.

"What Are My Goals?"

At fifty years of age we are not merely something that technology can chew up and spit out, are we? We have our own goals, don't we? Well, if this is true, think of four work goals you have in mind for the next five years. You could only think of two? When you were twenty, you would have had a list as long as your arm. What happened? Where are all those personal benchmarks you used to have: to be a $35,000-a-year man, to be president of the company, plant foreman, a full professor, to get the East Coast territory?

In the past, our goals were our beacons. We awoke at 5:00 A.M. and bolted out of the house on our way to hustle a new client. Some goals were short-term, some were long-term, but they were all goals that gave us direction, accomplishment, and identity at work.

But where are our goals today? Today we seem apathetic, more of a commodity than a creator of goals. Fears of obsolescence and overspecialization and "I've been moved" preclude us from setting new goals, preferring defensive driving or riding it out.

A loss of goals can be caused from either arriving too soon at our goal or never quite making it. Many of us set goals in early life and find that, through luck or competence, we attain them quite early in mid-life. A large number of metapausal men find they strove to "be somebody someday," only to wonder "if that's all there is."

It is important that the middle-aged man understand why he feels that the "wind is out of his sails," why he doesn't give so much of a damn about his work any more, and why, after all these years, he doesn't seem to have much energy and desire to keep clomping along.

"I've Got to Meet the Competition"

We also feel trapped because of the "good-guys-finish-last" philosophy. The free-enterprise system is "our system," but to the middle-aged man it can form an additional aspect of his entrapment. Take Willie Lohman again, explaining this phi-losophy to one of his sons:

That's just what I mean. Bernard can get the best marks in school, y'understand, but when he gets out in the business world, y'understand, you are going to be five times ahead of him. That's why I thank Almighty God you're both built like Adonises. Because the man who makes an appearance in the business world, the man who creates personal interest, is the man who gets ahead. Be liked and you will never want.

Taught to get the best grades, excel on the varsity track team, and be at the top of his class (or at least get credit for trying), the American male makes turning right at Oak Street the "big game" each day. Like a gladiator, he moves into a row of cars stacked up on the freeway on his way to meeting the competition in the Coliseum. Like Saturday's football hero, the small businessman tries to get up for the game plan. But old forty-eight is tired. It's been a long season, and he wonders if "killing the competition" is "where it's at" (to borrow his son's term). Each year, he turns the clock back and starts over: a new quota, more sales, more clients, a bigger market.

As one middle-aged man said:

I'd like to feel that when I'm approaching 50–55 that I'm still wanted by Autoline, not tossed on the rubbish heap. With the time and energy I've put in, it would be a crying shame if my past efforts were not appreciated when I start slowing down.[14]

Old number forty-eight's problems with the competition do not come only from the outside competition. He competes inside the company, with his rival for advancement.

Most forty- to fifty-year-old executives from the local grocery to the largest U.S. corporations today are caught in the gulf between career aspirations and reality, and in the abrupt narrowing that occurs near the top of the executive pyramid, the inside competition seems too much for the middle-aged man.

Our competitiveness often drives us without much compassion or caring: "Sorry, George, but we will be closing the accounting section now that the computer is in place." "Sorry, George, but we need to tighten our belts and we've selected Jim, a younger man." "Sorry, George, since our merger, we've been trying to think of what to do with you."

All of these forms of competition keep old number forty-eight on the treadmill, turning right at Oak Street each day.

"I'm Bored with My Work"

Another characteristic of entrapment in work that confuses the middle-aged man's "Who am I?" is that of routine.

Metathought introduces this topic to our minds: "Well, there's routine in everything," we might say. "I never minded it before." "The nine-to-five scene hasn't been that bad—until now." "Why am I so fussy about my routine?" "What's the matter with me?" This barrage of metathoughts is common in mid-life.

The white-collar man strives for variety in his work. In his early career, he was excited about not having any two days that are alike. Gradually he becomes a partial slave to the routine. This "doing-it-by-the-numbers" feeling was well expressed by a faculty colleague who stated during the first week of a new academic year, "Well, we only have thirty-two weeks left until graduation."

While it's true that man is a creature of habit, he also needs challenge and excitement. Middle-aged men, holding down the same job for three or more years, often feel like a fixture. Listen to the story Jack told his counseling group: "Not only does the routine bother me more, but I feel like a nonperson, part of automation. It's like the feeling you get on the freeway when you've driven a long, familiar stretch and can't actually remember driving it."

So, routine gets us. You stop at a local bar early one night to get away from the boredom of work, only to have a friend say, "What's new at work, Ed?" Your answer, "The same old stuff." In *Candide,* Voltaire states that work keeps us from three vices, one of which is boredom. Well, that might have been okay in France, but when the middle-aged man in modern industry feels the most exciting part of the week was playing poker with the numbers on his paycheck, something's wrong.

Perhaps we reject the "I've-been-moved" philosophy, feel overspecialzed and maybe a little out of date. And, further, if we lack goals and are tired of fighting the competition, then doesn't it seem that what we have left is the routine, the minutiae, the red tape? Research about routine and its characteristics bears out this conclusion. In a study of continuously performed tasks, men in their sixties were only about half as fast as men in their twenties. Another study found that monotonous tasks have an adverse effect and induce workers' alienation.[15]

After examining the elements of work entrapment within The Gray Itch, we should look at how many act out their entrapment.

"Let Me Out of Here"

Taking off for Aspen or drowning one's sorrows in booze are probably the most common ways of escaping, although mistresses, motorcycles, and Maseratis are not uncommon.

Escape from work—or avoidance behavior, as the psychologists call it—is a common reaction to the feeling of routine and entrapment in work. "A ticket to Tahiti, please—one way," you fantasize to yourself. Another metathought enters your consciousness: "I wonder how much those condominiums in Hawaii are." These comments relate to the *Gauguin syndrome* in many a middle-aged man. Gauguin, as you recall, left Paris for a new life on Tahiti—lush fruit, foliage, and *les femmes*. Well, at certain times all of us feel this need to escape, to turn left at Oak Street.

A panic sets in as we spend a restless night dreaming of being laid off, struggling for a new job, years of service and early retirement. We find it would be pretty hard to live on Oak Street on a pension of $500 a month. The panic also is fed by the thought that we could take "the great escape" but that must be discounted because of the 10½ percent mortgage on our home.

The panic is only partially lessened when we bolster ourselves by telling ourselves that we are the best vice-president in the industry, that we really are well known in our field, or that certainly another job would be possible. But starting all over again, all those years of conferences and lunches, discussions, sales meetings—starting over again is like an experiment and seems frightening.

"My Work Depresses Me These Days"

Common, too, is normal middle-aged depression, which comes on us suddenly. We stop momentarily on the assembly line or at our desk. We look out the window, look back to the pictures of our family, glance at the annual forecast before us, and a metathought occurs to us: "I'm stuck here."

This depression awakens us suddenly at night—we feel as though we've lost something. After hours of studying the ceiling or watching the light on the digital clock, we crawl further down into the blankets. Now depression has gripped us with fear, fear of our lack of control over these downers. Our inability to pull out of them preoccupies us. Regular incidents like these can cause the middle-aged businessman to develop a complex set of consequences ignited by that mild depression in the office. Take Jerry's sleepless night:

I just laid there, eyes wide open like Little Orphan Annie, staring at what I could make out of the pattern on the wallpaper. I couldn't stop thinking about where I was professionally and not even knowing where I wanted to be instead.

Kicking the Dog and the Wife

Another way to act out our sense of entrapment is to blame others. For those middle-aged button-down-collar types who overidentify with their work, a bad day can mean a loss of *self-*esteem; and we often take it out on the family.

Many wives can tell what kind of an evening it's going to be by the way the garage door closes. The kids head for their rooms, and the dog takes off under the bed. The wife takes a deep breath, opens the door, and says, "Hi, how was your day?" Take the reaction of Sally, a suburban Chicago housewife:

When it nears the time for Ted to come home, I can feel my stomach churn and my nerves tighten. It used to be I couldn't wait to see him. Now those first five seconds through the door, one look at his face, the way he says hello and puts down his briefcase, and I can predict exactly how the evening will play.

What does the middle-aged man expect of his family? It's incredible how a man can spend his twelve-hour day involved in time and territory analysis and think it's possible to compensate for that rotten twelve-hour day between 9:00 and 10:30 P.M. at night with his family. Listen to Mary's story about her husband, Marv's, false expectation:

I just don't know what he wants anymore. The kids up or the kids put to bed, a hot dinner or something light, an evening with my company or alone, staring into the aquarium. I'm not sure if anything I can do even matters at this point.

How can 20 percent of his "Who am I?" (family or other) compensate for 60 percent of his identity (work) after a bad day? Notice how we can't kick the boss, but we can sure throw our weight around at home.

Workaholic

While the middle-aged man "brings his work home" and dumps it on his family inappropriately, he can also take his work entrapment more seriously and "bury himself in his work." Compensating as he does, a twelve-hour day becomes a fifteen-hour one, and business trips carry over into the weekend. He becomes one of those who hasn't seen his backyard in the daylight since last summer's barbecue.

"The Hell with the Establishment"

The nonconformist at work is often a talented and experienced guy who, because of his feelings of entrapment, acts out the antagonist role. At the staff meeting, if consensus is near, he brings up a new point. In hopes the people at work *won't* understand, he wears a turquoise choker to an important meeting. If a ten-minute coffee break is common, he takes thirty minutes. Within him a new identity emerges—the detached antagonist, the critic.

Years of being "a member of the team" juxtaposed with today's entrapment gives him cause to "do his own thing." It's amazing how he gets so much attention by being different. "I should have started this twenty years earlier," his subconscious tells him. He doesn't need goals or to concern himself with overspecialization. He is himself a new specialty.

Acting out by escape, booze, depression, or kicking the dog, the man at metacenter insulates his identity and ego from further damage through work entrapment. All of these so-called ways out only seem that way; in actuality they add to further alienation at work and from himself.

Rewinding the Career Clock

One last area of entrapment in work needs mentioning. When one gets out of synchronization with his career clock, he soon feels further trapped and more confused about who he is. Middle-aged men seem to have a predetermined schedule on their career clocks. States of satisfaction are reported as, "I'm about where I should be at this time in my career." While others less satisfied with their timetable report, "I lost a lot of time in my two previous jobs," or "If only I knew then what I know now, I would have moved further in the company."

David Glover, a finance broker, states:

There have been many times of personal questioning about my

occupation. The worst time came when I approached the magic mark of 40. During that time, we were in the heart of a bear market and this is a highly emotional business.[16]

We have examined the dilemma of work in mid-life—the middle-aged man's overidentification with who he is within his job. After many years of punching the clock, this dilemma turns into a sense of entrapment in middle age. Feeling trapped by his mobility, possible obsolescence, and overspecialization, the middle-aged metapausal man adds fear to his sense of entrapment. Competition in and out of the office, lack of goals, a career clock out of whack, and routine all lead to boredom.

Rapid-fire metathoughts cause him to act out his Gray Itch in certain ways. Escape through dropping out, alcohol, kicking the wife and dog, becoming a nonconformist, or being depressed are important factors in the work life of the middle-aged man, 60 to 80 percent of who he is.

H.I.M.M.
(Hallberg Index of Male Metapause)

VICE PRESIDENT WHO?

The statements that follow should represent some of your present and future feelings and concerns about your work as discussed in this chapter.

DIRECTIONS

Please mark each statement twice. First, mark with a circle one number for each statement to represent your nearest current feeling about the subject. Second, mark one number with a square to represent where you wish to be regarding the statement. Higher numbers should equal stronger feelings.

EXAMPLE

I hate to lose to the
competition.   1   2   ③   4   5   ⑥   7   8   9   10

WORK CONTINUA

1. My career is at a very crucial point.
   1 2 3 4 5 6 7 8 9 10

2. I feel uncertain about my work.
   1 2 3 4 5 6 7 8 9 10

3. I can see the end of the road in the company.
   1 2 3 4 5 6 7 8 9 10

4. I don't feel my work is important in my life.
   1 2 3 4 5 6 7 8 9 10

5. If I were thirty-five again, I wouldn't feel so trapped.
   1 2 3 4 5 6 7 8 9 10

6. With my age and experience, it would be easy to find another job in my field.
   1 2 3 4 5 6 7 8 9 10

7. If my boss retired, I would like his job.
   1 2 3 4 5 6 7 8 9 10

8. I seem to be a loner at work these days.
   1 2 3 4 5 6 7 8 9 10

9. I never think of retirement.
   1 2 3 4 5 6 7 8 9 10

10. I wish I were freer to be my own boss.
    1 2 3 4 5 6 7 8 9 10

11. I find I'm overspe-   1 2 3 4 5 6 7 8 9 10
    cialized at work.

12. I'm one of the best   1 2 3 4 5 6 7 8 9 10
    in my field.

13. I feel my knowledge   1 2 3 4 5 6 7 8 9 10
    about work is up to
    date.

14. I need to find a small 1 2 3 4 5 6 7 8 9 10
    store or business
    somewhere.

15. It's hard for me to   1 2 3 4 5 6 7 8 9 10
    recall major work
    accomplishments
    for the last year.

16. I'm self-propelled in 1 2 3 4 5 6 7 8 9 10
    my work these days.

17. I enjoy beating   1 2 3 4 5 6 7 8 9 10
    the competition in
    the marketplace.

18. The competition   1 2 3 4 5 6 7 8 9 10
    from inside, from
    my peers, is greater
    than that from the
    outside.

19. I live to work.   1 2 3 4 5 6 7 8 9 10

20. I feel that my work is 1 2 3 4 5 6 7 8 9 10
    getting in the way of
    other things I want
    to do.

21. When somebody asks me what's new at work, I always answer, "Nothing."   1 2 3 4 5 6 7 8 9 10

22. Routine doesn't bother me.   1 2 3 4 5 6 7 8 9 10

23. I have a lot of trouble understanding criticism of my work.   1 2 3 4 5 6 7 8 9 10

24. I'd like to spend the rest of my career settled in the place I presently live.   1 2 3 4 5 6 7 8 9 10

SCORING

Now add up the total sum of your circled numbers and squared numbers and enter them below:

○ Circled Score _____   ☐ Squared Score: _____

A comparison of your scores can be obtained in two steps:

1. Compare your own current and wished for scores on each statement.
2. If a difference of more than twenty points exists between your *total* current and wished for scores, refer to the corresponding Metacare Guidelines in Chapter 12.

Chapter 5

THE PHYSICAL ME

One of the major facets of "Who am I?" for the middle-aged man is his physical self. From flexing his biceps in front of the mirror while in junior high to smashing that tennis ball in his 40s, a man's physical self gives messages about "who he is."

Remember how you could drink a case of beer and ski hard the next day? Remember how you felt when you hit that 250-yard drive or took off your shirt at the We-Don't-Tell Motel? Remember how warming up for an athletic event was just that, and not a precheck to see if all the parts were working?

But today, as in other areas of "Who am I?," metathoughts are heard: "Why am I out of breath?" "Boy, it's cold in this meeting." "My legs feel like spaghetti." An important researcher on mid-life, Bernice Neugarten, says:

The most dramatic cues for the middle-aged man are often biological. The increased attention centered upon his health, the decrease in the efficiency of his body, the death of friends of the same age—these are common signs that prompt many men to describe bodily changes as the most salient characteristic of middle-age.[1]

One middle-aged man points out, "It was the sudden heart attack of a friend that made the difference." Another says, "I realized I could no longer count on my body as I used to. My body is now unpredictable."

Common metathoughts about our bodies indicate two areas

that need exploration. First, what about some of the natural physical changes that occur in mid-life, such as those in metabolism, hair, skin, senses, hormones, heart, and memory. And second, what are some of the common physical and psychological maladies that unfortunately beset some of us, such as stress, depression, arthritis, alcoholism, and diseases of the heart and prostate?

Body Geography in Mid-Life

Here we are interested in the normal, healthy body and some of the conditions that change within it; only minor emphasis will be put on diseases in mid-life. While the chapter is extensive, don't feel that all middle-aged men suffer from all that is presented. Besides, you could be older.

"Everything I Eat Turns to Fat"

Fat is one of the important distortions of our bodies in middle life, and is the cause of many metathoughts. If you think this isn't true, go try on your high school letterman's sweater. If you are like the rest of us, your letterman's stripes are up around your shoulders and the buttons stick out like prunes on the front of a snowman.

In the last twenty or thirty years, you've gained two inches on your belt, an inch on your collar and probably twenty pounds. The ballooning of our bodies is caused mainly by overeating, overdrinking, and metabolic changes. Do you sanctimoniously pass up breakfast and lunch, only to eat sixty Ritz crackers with your four martinis in the evening? When you're out to dinner, are you more interested in the menu than your delicious date? All of these are common horizontal, expansionist characteristics of the middle-aged man.

Not only does fat dominate the wide-angle lens camera used for your twenty-fifth high-school reunion picture, but often other subtle body distortions occur due to fat. After three hours in your new suit, do the pants look like hip-huggers? And does your tailor stutter as he asks you, "Where do you wear your pants?" You think, "To work or play." What he *wants* to ask is, "Where is your waist?" And isn't it true our horizontal growth has made important manly parts appear relatively smaller as our upper bodies explode in size?

Calories can change our thoughts about ourselves. The reasons for weight gain in mid-life actually need little description. Mainly, it is our own inability to adjust to a *new problem* in our lives. The problem is a simple one: as we age, we require less food to maintain our somewhat deteriorating bodies. Literally, cells decay. Metabolism slows and physical activity lessens. This decrease in need for food occurs when we sit on our tails for at least an eight-hour day, or on that power mower as we buzz around our front lawns on Saturday morning.

Isn't it incredible how we complain about fat and yet our belt size increases along with the number of candles on our birthday cakes? And isn't it interesting how we seem to consume three drinks at lunch (400 calories), four drinks before dinner (600), and maybe that small sherry before bed (250)? Enough calories (1,250 without olives, tonic, or cherries) to keep a small boy active on a playground for half a day. Of *course* we diet—salad (100 calories) with Roquefort (300 calories); veal (300) cordon bleu (400); low-cal hamburger (200) with béarnaise sauce (300). There are also those countless hors d'oeuvre and the box of Wheat Thins that reminds us of the cookie jar of our childhood.

And now that we can afford those fancy French restaurants with their soufflés and mousses, we see ourselves putting on the dog and pounds at the same time. Worse yet, we can put on weight, yet write it off.

Still another characteristic of obesity (and one that may motivate some of us to cut down on food intake) is that *overeating,* like overdrinking, can have a definite effect on the reduction of our sexual interests. Are you concerned *now?*

Mid-life must be countered with a reduction of food intake; otherwise, our belt size will surpass our age. Just think of being fifty-eight years old.

"I Wonder How Much a Hair Transplant Costs?"

Isn't it terrible that hair is such a mark of youth and manhood? From Samson to Prince Valiant to the quarterback fading back for a pass with golden locks protruding out of his helmet, hair has traditionally symbolized an important quality of manhood. Unfortunately, most of us have to pay our barber twenty dollars in mid-life to compensate for its loss with a design that combs our sideburns over the tops of our heads.

Or if we are fortunate enough to have a good head of hair, a gray weed patch often threatens to take over the crop. Remember the day your thirteen-year-old said, "Dad, have you ever heard of Grecian Formula 16?" Or after a tough day you relax before the TV, only to see a commercial with your favorite baseball star of the fifties, Bob Feller—yes, Bob Feller— promoting a before-and-after hair-dye job.

What happened to that beautiful head of hair that took twenty minutes to comb into a pompadour when you were in high school? You say, "It doesn't matter much." Your wife says, "Baldness is sexy." However, it bothers you. Why else would you put on your hat first when you get dressed in the morning, or tell people you've worn your hair off on the headboard of your bed because of your sexuality? It is disconcerting to wait a week for an appointment for that twenty-dollar hairstyle and have your barber say, after five minutes in the chair, "Well, that's it"—and you know he's right. What really happens to this all-important sign of male virility and body ego?

"Being Bald Is Sexy"

Our hair grows at the rate of about a half an inch a month and often lives from about two to four years; then new hairs replace the lost ones (for some of us). Most important is the papilla at the lower end of the hair follicle that contains the blood supply and the nerve endings that are needed for the growth of the hair. Our hair continues to grow as long as the papilla provides nourishment and new cells regenerate at the base of the hair root. The cause of the permanent loss of hair is unknown, but some feel it relates to degeneration of cells at the hair root.

"Gray Hair Is Dashing"

Being a Silver Fox might be nice for some, but for most of us it's a constant reminder of Father Time. Girls we meet say, "Sir ... I like your gray hair. It looks so distinguished." But it's still gray. Hair produced during our early lives is color-primed by the production of pigment, like a new Ford. But for some reason (yet unknown), in mid-life pigment production slows down, causing gray.

Some of us gray at our temples first, while others' beards whiten first. Regardless, it doesn't pay to pluck out those first gray ones, for the crop will continue to grow without your thinning. The irony is that as the top of our heads become more exposed to the elements, through loss of hair, hair on other parts of our body seems to increase—on our backs, in our ears and noses.

So, the Prince Valiant days are over, and our relative victory over baldness is compensated only by our gray hair swept up by the barber's broom.

"My Skin Looks Like Yesterday's Balloon"

Some days we look at those once-supple arms and smooth skin and think of a half-deflated tether ball or yesterday's carnival balloon. Unfortunately, as we age, our skin and its elasticity undergo change. Sometimes this old-leather look seems to come on us quite fast. R. Hill informs us, "Degenerative changes frequently become apparent in the fourth decade of life and may appear even earlier in persons who have been exposed continuously to the elements." [2] What generally happens is that the "oil can" glands of the skin secrete less lubricant and the skin dries and loses some of its elasticity. This, coupled with a natural loss of muscle and fat tissues, can make middle-aged skin look like a used grocery bag.

Another phenomenon of the skin in mid-life is liver spots. Liver spots are increases in pigmentation of the epidermis (outer layer of skin). Solid substances, such as pigments, become deposited within and between the cells. It's like your furnace when it gets choked with cinders and can't maintain a good fire. These spots usually appear on the back of the hands, or on the side of the neck or face. Generally, they don't occur on skin that is usually protected by clothing, indicating that sunlight and weather might add to the middle-aged man's susceptibility to liver spots.

So, alas, we are subject to yet another paradox: the pigmentation leaves our hair and collects on our necks, faces, ears, or the backs of our hands.

In mid-life, our skin has more of a tendency to flush, due to vasomotor disturbances in the body mechanism. This means, in exercise or embarrassment, the opening and closing of the arteries or veins to accommodate the blood is a little slower. Remember how blotchy you were the last time you were mad at your wife, or embarrassed on your birthday?

"Am I Having a Hot Flash?"

Certain metathoughts occur to some of us: "What's wrong with me?" "I have to start buying a better brand of whiskey." "Am I having a hot flash?" There is some evidence that, as we age, our *skin* thins out, not our blood. When our wives say that we have "thin skin," it's true in more ways than one. Our thermostat tends to decrease in size as we age. As these sensors atrophy, we tend to lose our insulation and feel chilly more often.

From Cold to Hot

Or the opposite happens: that feeling comes over us quickly and we ask our bed partners to throw off the blankets or our business partners to throw open a window during a board meeting. What happens is, our computer increases our blood supply to surface parts to compete with the warmer environment, such as after exercise, and an extra supply of blood diffuses through our system as the capillaries dilate. The message here to our system is "Reduce body temperature." The opposite is also true: We are cold, the capillaries constrict. However, as we mentioned, in mid-life our thermostats sometimes get out of whack, and even without exercise, our capillaries dilate, so we go around asking everybody, "Are you cold?" or "It's hot in here, isn't it?" to verify some of our own internal weather forecasts.

It follows, then, if our thermostat or sensors get stuck, other systems must take over—and with a thermostat we can't hit or cuss at, perspiration takes over, giving us an overkill on our brow or under our arms. At times, the crazy thermostat says 80 when it's only 42. So we sweat at coffee breaks and have chills at the annual meeting. One researcher comments:

Age changes and temperature regulation have been observed in industrial workers: For instance, in older miners who sweat less when they are working and more when they are resting, because the sweating and circulating mechanisms are sluggish and no longer capable of the same range of reaction.[3]

"Can I Blame It on Metabolism?"

Much of our change in hot and cold is caused by one of our greatest body mysteries, metabolism. The basal metabolism rate is defined as "the calories one consumes while at rest." Our metabolic rate increases with exercise or excitement but also declines with age. It is estimated that a sixty-five-year-old would need to walk nine miles to burn off the calories he could have burned sitting in a chair all day at twenty years of age. This decline is caused primarily by a decrease in the total number of cells, less activity in the major regions of the body, such as the liver and the muscles, and a slowing of thyroid secretions.

Our metabolism does change and it does cause us certain problems. Some adjustments need to be made when it comes to eating, drinking, and exercise. Slower metabolism results in fewer calories burned. If food intake and exercise don't change during mid-life, we may still gain weight due to a saggy metabolism.

"My Wife Has Hormone Problems—Not Me"

We have all heard about the hormonal changes in the *note* female, such as an estrogen decrease. However, few men know how the male hormone system changes in the amount and balance of androgens secreted.

The hormones of our system are basically its primer, its choke on cold mornings. Several types of hormones are part of a family called androgens. Within the pituitary gland, located at the base of the brain, two hormones are born. The first, LH (lutein hormone), produces testosterone. Testosterone helps develop maleness in adolescence—that beard, that deep voice, the Charles Atlas build. The second hormone, FSH (follicle-stimulating hormones), helps in the production of sperm. These hormones and their production are monitored by the hypothalamus. It is generally accepted that the production of testosterone increases progressively from the ages of ten to fourteen, reaching its highest point between twenty-two and twenty-five and maintaining its level for about ten years.

Testosterone decreases in middle age seem to cause the loss of physical stamina as well, according to Drs. M. Prados and B. Ruddick.[4] It declines gradually. This decline is most obvious and rapid between the ages of forty and fifty, and, at the age of sixty, androgen production returns to the prepuberty level.

In metapause, hormone decreases are controlled by the hypothalamus, which also happens to be one of the centers related to depression, stress, and anxiety. Though conclusive data are lacking, some evidence indicates that decreases in our hormone output cause behavioral changes related to depression.

So You, Too, May Have a Cycle

One of the common symptoms of metapause is a set of roller-coaster psychological highs and lows that could relate to changes in hormone secretions. Estelle Ramey reported in 1972 that certain mood shifts occurred with the change in hormone production. Her study of private transport companies in Japan found that bus routes and schedules were adjusted to maximize efficiency and minimize accidents among bus drivers on the basis of their "time of the month." Also, a report from United Airlines indicates that adjustment of pilots' schedules on a regular basis due to shifts in biorhythms may be a common occurrence.

It has also been estimated that men have a four- to six-week cycle of mood comparable to those of women. While evidence of mood comparables is not complete, male hormonal secretion cycles may be responsible for cyclical variations in men's moods. Ramey also found in a study of factory workers that "their emotions varied on a near-monthly cycle; low periods were characterized by apathy, indifference or a tendency to magnify minor problems all out of proportion; high periods were often marked by a feeling of well-being, energy and low body-weight and a decreased need for sleep." [5] Although the exact relationship between biorhythms and metapause is unknown, Soddy reports one study that showed "men had individual cycles of (sexual) activity, and fluctuations tended to be accentuated in middle age." [6] A male cycle of three weeks was suggested but not confirmed.

It appears our moods may be regulated by hormonal production, which in turn appears to have some biothythmic cycle. A recent *Psychology Today* article says that our bio-rhythm system is related to the luteinizing hormones which affect sex hormones.[7]

"I Feel Bushed Half the Time"

At metacenter, physical or psychological fatigue interrupts the sense of well-being and seems to last all day on occasion. At its maximum in our twenties and thirties, studies indicate that our physical energy decreases from then on. These changes are often due to muscular loss, decreased cardiac output, and less efficient respiration. "Testosterone (hormone) decrease seems to add to the loss of physical stamina," report researchers Prados and Ruddick.[8] But fatigue and boredom are closely tied together. Some evidence indicates "not getting up" psychologically may feel the same to us as physical fatigue.

Fatigue obviously not only affects one's physical self in general, but can change the sexual appetite. Masters and Johnson report:

Fatigue is an important element in the involution of male sexuality and exerts an ever-increasing influence during and beyond middle age. Mental as well as physical fatigue seems to take its toll here. Extensive physical activity in recreational interests and work interests demands can cause fatigue which may influence sexual performance.[9]

One forty-four-year-old told me of his sexual interest and fatigue, "Of course I'm not as young as I used to be. But it isn't so much the loss of sexual interest. I think it's more an energy factor." He continued, "I think as the years go by, you have less sexual desire. In fact, when you are younger, there is a need in addition to the desire. I still enjoy sex, but not with the fervor of youth. Not because I've lost my feelings for my wife, but because it happens to you physically."

"I'm as Strong as I Ever Was"

Unfortunately, if the superjock feels all he needs to do to return to his youthful body is run an extra mile, he's off the mark. General cell and system deterioration do occur *gradually* as we age.

To be sure, exercise and good diet may keep us up to date, but that date is not 1949. We can't turn the clock back. Besides, who wants acne again or the back seat of a '49 Chevy?

"My Teeth Are Beginning to Cost Me More Than the Country Club"

If you thought your auto payments were high, look at your yearly dental payments over the last few years. And I don't mean the braces for the kids. I am talking about the inlays and onlays, root canals, gum repairs, and extractions. One of the common physical changes within the middle-aged man is in his teeth. At metacenter, gums begin to recede and teeth begin to yellow because of the thickening of secondary dentine. There is also a reduction of saliva, which may increase decay.

"Here's Looking at You" (The Eyes Had It)

Several aspects of vision decline as we approach middle age and beyond. These include distance vision, adaptation to darkness, and near vision. The ability to see clearly at a distance remains fairly constant until forty-five or fifty, and then declines only gradually. Our ability to see clearly when lights are low diminishes in middle age because light has a harder time penetrating the thickened lens and cornea. Focusing on near objects decreases at a constant rate between the ages of fifty and sixty and accounts for the need for reading glasses or bifocals in middle age.

The eye lens begins to age as early as infancy. It becomes more opaque and less elastic in our middle years because it continues to grow without shedding older cells. The gradual atrophy of nerve cells and a poorer blood supply also contribute to impaired vision in middle age. The yellowing of the lens causes our color sensitivity to show a gradual loss of fine discrimination.

"I Wonder How the Old Ticker Is?"

While we hear a lot about the possible diseases of the heart, most men at metacenter know little about what a healthy heart looks or feels like. The heart changes, but not dramatically, in mid-life. For example, the heart changes little in weight relative to other organs in normal aging.

After the age of fifty or so, the heart rate gradually becomes slower and more irregular due to the decrease in demand we place on it. And skipping a beat can be more common.

Certainly, activity is an important consideration for the beating heart. If your other muscles are degenerating because all you lift is a pen, should your heart react differently? Hours and days of sitting flat in your chair at the office or at home can lead to an inefficient heart. After all, look what happens to your golf swing between summer and the company tournament in March. Even during sexual activity many metapausal men concern themselves with their hearts.

Dr. H. L. Karpman descusses sex and activity even after a coronary:

No, sex really isn't that much of a strain. For a middle-aged patient who's had a heart attack, during sexual activity, the heart averages 117 beats a minute. But it can go as high as 144 beats a minute—about the energy expenditure of climbing a flight of stairs.[10]

The healthy middle-aged man can't afford to live out his life with a heart-attack phobia that translates each gas pain into a potential coronary.

"My I.Q. Has Really Slipped"

"Well, even if my body is aging, I'm sure a lot sharper than those dumb kids at work," you might say. Are you? At least four types of intelligence do exist. According to Paul Baltes and

K. Warner Schaie, it appears that we decline only in one of the four measures as we age—thank goodness!

The first area of intelligence is crystalized intelligence. This comprises skills acquired through education and growing up in a particular culture, such as language, numerical skills, and inductive reasoning.

A second type of intelligence is cognitive flexibility, which measures the ability to shift from one way of thinking to another in familiar intellectual operations. An example is when one must provide either an antonym or a synonym to a word, depending on whether a word appears in capital or lower-case letters.

The third type of intelligence is visual-motor flexibility, which measures a similar but independent skill that is involved in shifting from familiar to unfamiliar patterns in tasks requiring coordination between visual and motor abilities, such as when one copies words but interchanges capitals with lower-case letters.

The fourth type is visualization, which measures the ability to organize and process visual materials. This involves tasks such as finding a simple figure contained in a complex one or identifying a picture that is incomplete.

Of the four, it appears that only the visual-motor flexibility is impaired with age. In a recent article in *Psychology Today,* Baltes and Schaie stated:

> There is no strong age-related change in cognitive flexibility, for the most important dimension, crystalized intelligence and for visualization as well, we see a systematic increase in scores for various age groups, right into age 70. Even people over 70 improve from their first testing to the second.[11]

In fact, these same researchers were able to improve the response speed of elderly persons rather dramatically. The results indicated that subjects who were trained in improving their skills raised subsequent I.Q. scores.

In certain other research on intelligence tests that have not isolated speed as a factor there does seem to be a decline of intelligence with age. In the Wechsler Adult Intelligence Scale, this seems to be true.[12] From about the age of 30 or so, there is a gradual reduction of intelligence scores into mid-life and a continuous one thereafter.

As we age, other factors affect our use of our minds. We tend to narrow our interests and are less apt to explore and learn in new areas, like the businessman who thought brainstorming techniques had to end in a yes-or-no answer. We also tend to fall back on our experience. We tend to restrict our natural processes to only a single answer. As we age, we tend to be less experimental in our approaches to problem solving and conceptualizing. This overall rigidity reduces certain kinds of intelligence. Part of the problem of I.Q. score reduction lies in the different way our memories work.

"You Remember Old What's-His-Name"

This brings us to another common mid-life problem area: memory. Several factors need mention.

Beyond any doubt, the size and weight of the brain decreases as we age. Along with a general reduction, we are all aware of how hardening of the arteries and alcohol may reduce the number of brain cells even further.

Beyond the simple loss of memory, other factors must be kept in mind. Maybe the reason we can't remember "Old What's-His-Name" is that we have met so many Jims, Georges, and Eds in our lifetime. There is a common learning problem at any age: the psychological concepts of similarity and transfer of training. If two things we have learned are too similar, we are less able to transfer names and concepts to new situations. We may not have lost our faculties, but our computers may be overloaded.

Another interesting area—eh—where were we? ... Oh, yes, another interesting area relates to time frames—past, present, and future. In mid-life, certain shifts occur. Two patterns seem common: First, there is Larry, who has always looked ahead, riding like a star in his company. In his mid-forties, he realizes someday he will come to the end of the road. He shifts from a future time orientation to a past one. His favorite sentences begin: "When I was your age . . ." or "People don't work like they used to. . . ." Old Larry likes routine more than adventure. His past orientation allows him to relate in exact detail how the company did its accounting in 1954, but he can't for the life of him remember the figures in next year's forecast. A straight-line projection will place Larry into early old age and not unlike Grandma, who may have some difficulty knowing where she is on any one day but is able to describe what she wore to the junior prom on June 4, 1902, from 9:00 P.M. to 1:00 A.M.

Then, there's Bill. His realization that life is finite doesn't push his memory into the past, but he drops it into the present. Like the youth of the sixties, he wants "freedom now." He lives on "now time." His "you-don't-live-forever" attitude makes him unconcerned with his past and his future. He programs his memory to the present like Rod McKuen, who once said he only remembers the people he's met in the last few days.

We can see, then, that memory loss, particularly in middle life, may be largely a redirection of our retrieval systems. These physical changes represent the price we pay for being successful in mid-life, right?

Few can avoid the last pages as a map of their changing bodies. But most of us do avoid the maladies expressed in the next few pages—the second kind of change in our physical geography.

"What's a Prostate Problem?"

One of the subjects of preoccupation in the fifty-year-old male is his prostate. This Ping-Pong ball–sized gland can be a cause of important changes in his life, including his sex life. Located in the lower abdomen at the base of the urinary bladder, the prostate wraps around the urethra, the tube through which both urine and semen are expelled. Throughout life, the prostate's job is to produce certain elements in semen other than sperm.

As we age, the size of the prostate increases, but not significantly. After forty, certain changes do occur. Smooth muscle or connective tissue within the prostate increases, causing the prostate to soften. Often in the sixth decade of life the prostate is slightly enlarged and can cause a light urinary hesitation and a sense of fullness in the bladder. Take Steve. He gets up three times a night, but does little when he gets there.

After the age of forty, three diseases of the prostate may occur: chronic prostasis, often symptomatized by painful and/or premature ejaculation; nodular hyperphasia; and cancer. The prostate is the third most common site of cancer in men over fifty-five years of age.

The exact reason for the appearances of disease of the prostate in mid-life are still unknown, but it does appear to be linked to the decrease in hormones from the pituitary gland and testes.

Several old wives' tales exist about our changing prostates, most relating to our inability to perform sexually. While certain pain may occur in ejaculation and/or erection due to a serious prostate problem (not to be confused with problems of sexual overuse), there is no evidence that having prostate difficulties leads to impotence. Doctors theorize that most impotence occurring even after as uncommon an operation as a prostatectomy is more closely related to the loss of general sexual *interest* than the operation itself.

"I'll Just Have One More for the Road"

A few belts on the way home or at a neighbor's Saturday night party may be okay, but the Achilles' heel of the middle-aged man is alcohol.

Why are we so vulnerable to alcohol? Several hypotheses are possible: first, metapause; second, the gradual buildup over the years of being comfortable with half a snootful gives us an artificial sense of well-being—much like the wife of a middle-aged colleague who did not know her husband drank until he came home sober one night.

As our hormone production varies in mid-life, we begin to suffer the slings and arrows of depression and inflation. When we feel depressed, we have one more for the commute home. Unfortunately, alcohol in any large quantities is a depressant, and we start a depression spiral.

Beyond any doubt, excessive alcohol causes secondary impotence. It can also cause frigidity in women. After an initial failure in bed due to an evening of martinis, burgundy, and stingers, we panic. Metathoughts such as "I'm over the hill" or "I'm losing it" fill our minds until the next time. We fortify ourselves even more for the next bedtime encounter, perhaps loosening up over a couple of bottles of wine. The result: we have loosened up too much!

Masters and Johnson hold: "Secondary impotence developing in the male in the late 40's or early 50's has a higher incidence of direct association with excessive alcohol consumption than with any other single factor." [13] Unfortunately, few men see this as a direct cause of their impotence.

Perhaps one of the best-known effects of chronic alcohol abuse is its toll on the liver. Cirrhosis ranks ninth among the causes of death in the country and fourth among men over the age of forty. Cirrhosis is a common condition that causes some middle-aged men to appear to list to the left because of an oversized liver on the right. This swollen organ on the right side will gradually be converted to scar tissue in the alcoholic. (Yes, like that scar tissue around your knee caused by that old football injury.)

Common to the middle-aged man who belts more than his share is the dehydrating effect of alcohol and its counterpart, bloating. While alcohol promotes dehydration, this happens only as long as the blood alcohol level is increasing. Once the blood alcohol level plateaus, peaks, or declines, bloating occurs. The dehydrating effect of alcohol is lessened because alcohol enhances the retention of salts in the system due to sodium reabsorption.

Impotence and cirrhosis are not the only problems faced by the excessive drinker. Gastritis is another problem. Here the alcohol burns the stomach lining, causing a loss of appetite or "morning sickness" on an empty stomach in the morning. Vomiting may occur, and as the perennial Virgil Parks cartoon expresses, we feel like shaving our tongues instead of our faces in the morning.

Thus, it appears alcohol offers a special problem for the middle-aged man. It is true that "you only go around once," and if it's not your liver, it might be an ulcer from the pressure. If you want to advance yourself into senility at an ever-increasing rate, heavy boozing will do it.

Heart Disease

Two important heart maladies or diseases can occur in mid-life. These are hypertensive heart and coronary arteriosclerosis. A hypertensive heart, while usually a disease of old age, may begin in mid-life. Hypertensive persons often show an enlargement of the left ventricle of the heart.

With or without heart failure, electrocardiographs actually show signs of heart strain and enlargement from hypertension. Albert I. Lancing has reported, "Many patients begin both systolic and diastolic hypertension starting in middle life and extending well beyond the 60's before the termination of life, which is usually on a cardiovascular basis from heart failure.[14]

The kidneys also play an important part in the hypertensive heart. The higher one's blood pressure, the more the kidneys become diseased and the worse hypertension becomes. The author of the popular book *Relaxation Response* tells us:

In the normal kidney, if blood pressure decreases to low levels, the kidneys secrete hormone substances that increase blood pressure. The kidneys act as sensors to maintain adequate blood pressure. If a minimal amount of arteriosclerosis develops in the blood vessels of the kidneys, it will decrease the amount of blood flow to these organs, and the kidneys will become shrunken. The blocked kidney vessel leads to lower pressure within the kidney and this organ responds in turn by secreting hormones that raise blood pressure throughout the body.[15]

Coronary arteriosclerosis is the second most common heart malady in mid-life or beyond. It is commonly tied to high blood pressure caused by hypertension. In *Relaxation Response* it is also reported that there appears to be a genuine connection between arteriosclerosis and increased blood pressure and cholesterol.

Many serious cases of coronary heart disease are born in our forties. These cases are characteristically found in those over-weight males who have a high degree of musculature and those with a great deal of endomorphic fat buildup. There may be a lesson here for many of us.

Hardening of the arteries, or arteriosclerosis, increases in frequency and severity as age increases from about 30 years, with the ages between 50 and 70 showing the greatest mortality. It's like sending water through rusty pipes. The difference in pressure between a ¾-inch plastic pipe you put in your front lawn years ago and a ½-inch pipe was substantial, wasn't it? Well, an analogy can be made with your blood and arteries.

Diet, exercise, tension, family disposition, and heredity can vary the size of the pipes. Cholesterol and its causes can make a normal middle-aged heart look worse than a turn-of-the-century well spout.

"I Really Get Uptight"

Major stress for the middle-aged man is caused by events that upset the sequence and rhythm of life. Some of the major upsets in mid-life are family warfare, meeting the competition, pursuing a girl friend, and fearing old age.

Defining stress is almost impossible, but like the hives, it causes changes all over our bodies. These include increased supplies from the adrenal glands, where the regulation of body fluids and salts is maintained, and changes in blood pressure.

Stress not only affects the balance of our biological functions, it may also cause major illness in mid-life. Dr. Thomas Holmes and Dr. Richard Rahe developed a social readjustment rating scale following the hypothesis that the stress of losing your job, death of a parent, divorce, or many of the events common in mid-life can be scaled and given points. The more changes one undergoes in a year, the more likely one is to have a concomitant major health change. Dr. Rahe studied the illness pattern of 2,500 officers and enlisted men aboard Navy ships and found that 30 percent of the men with higher life-change scores developed nearly 90 percent of the illnesses during the first month of the cruise.[16]

The normal changes in our six-million-dollar metapausal man can be centered in a changing "Physical me," an important aspect of who we are. Subtle body-ego changes can lead to self-misunderstanding. Countless metathoughts regarding our fat, loss of hair or breath tend to confuse us. Being trapped within our aging bodies can cause as much stress, strain, and confusion on the part of the metapausal man as his changing work role, sexual life, or role within his family.

But don't despair—the average middle-aged man can expect to live for about another twenty-five years. He is still in a relatively high point of his life cycle. D. B. Bromley feels:

It finds the individual in a fairly good state of health; his psychological capacities are relatively unimpaired, and he has accumulated considerable experience which he can use to advantage at work, or in public or domestic affairs. He is as (financially) well off, secure and privileged as he is ever likely to be.[17]

The metapausal man is physically changing. His perceptions of himself are correct. Basic changes should not be dismissed, yet he doesn't need to count the nails in his coffin, either. Wishing yourself back on the varsity track team or projecting yourself into Social Security is not the answer. The answer lies in the understanding of *your* time and place and its strenghts and cautions.

H.I.M.M.
(Hallberg Index of Male Metapause)

PHYSICAL ME

The statements that follow should represent some of your present and future feelings and concerns about your physical self discussed in this chapter.

DIRECTIONS

Please mark each statement twice. First, mark with a circle one number for each statement to represent your nearest current feeling about the subject. Second, mark one number with a square to represent where you would wish to see yourself regarding the statement. Higher numbers should equal stronger feelings.

EXAMPLE

I need to slow down.   1 ② 3 4 5 6 ⑦ 8 9 10

PHYSICAL SELF CONTINUA

1. What's the use, the years will continue to take a lot out of me.   1 2 3 4 5 6 7 8 9 10

2. I really get out of breath.   1 2 3 4 5 6 7 8 9 10

3. I've got to slow down.   1 2 3 4 5 6 7 8 9 10

4. I wish I could lose some weight.   1 2 3 4 5 6 7 8 9 10

5. I occasionally do not feel like going to some event if it takes physical effort.
       1 2 3 4 5 6 7 8 9 10

6. I would be quite content to remain as old as I am now.
       1 2 3 4 5 6 7 8 9 10

7. I see the same guy I have always seen when I look in the mirror.
       1 2 3 4 5 6 7 8 9 10

8. I'm more forgetful these days.
       1 2 3 4 5 6 7 8 9 10

9. I drink less now than I once did.
       1 2 3 4 5 6 7 8 9 10

10. Sometimes when I drink I really get depressed.
       1 2 3 4 5 6 7 8 9 10

11. The tension is really getting to me.
       1 2 3 4 5 6 7 8 9 10

12. I really seem uptight lately.
       1 2 3 4 5 6 7 8 9 10

13. I could eat all day.
       1 2 3 4 5 6 7 8 9 10

14. I'm cold a lot of the time.
       1 2 3 4 5 6 7 8 9 10

15. My heart seems to skip a beat once in a while.
       1 2 3 4 5 6 7 8 9 10

16. My memory is not quite as good as it was.

                                     1 2 3 4 5 6 7 8 9 10

17. I often feel jittery.

                                     1 2 3 4 5 6 7 8 9 10

18. There are too many major changes in my life.

                                     1 2 3 4 5 6 7 8 9 10

19. Suddenly I feel down sometimes.

                                     1 2 3 4 5 6 7 8 9 10

20. I feel more like sex after a couple of drinks.

                                     1 2 3 4 5 6 7 8 9 10

SCORING

Now add up the sum total of your circled numbers and your squared numbers and enter them below:

◯ Circled score: _____ ☐ Squared Score:_____

A comparison of your scores can be obtained in two steps:

1. Compare your own current and wished for scores on each statement.
2. If a difference of more than twenty points exists between your *total* current and wished for scores, refer to the corresponding Metacare Guidelines in Chapter 12.

Chapter 6
YOUR SEXUAL I.D.

For the middle-aged man feeling his way into a dark bedroom at fifty, sex becomes his name, rank, and serial number. Men like you and I attempt to prove who we are by what's in our pants. In the past, our time in bed reaffirmed our machismo. Our sack time directly related to our marriage continuity. After all, the kids are the fruit of our loins, aren't they? Sexual encounters have always left us feeling virile, full of prowess. Isn't sex the way we evaluate our marriage?

For many in middle age, using sex to prove who they are can be confusing. Due to former conditioning—the numbers attached to sexual encounters—the *changing* middle-aged man develops a set of fears about his sexual adequacy. This results in additional identity confusion and questions about his manhood, another aspect of The Gray Itch.

The metapausal man is truly caught between the four-poster and the water bed. In mid-life we tend to compare our 1940s and 1950s conditioning of the past ("I shouldn't have gone all the way," or "I took advantage of her") with the swinger philosophy of today ("You wouldn't buy a car without driving it first, would you?"). Extraordinary shifts in our society from the good old days to newer days are with us, providing new sexual definitions of virility, promiscuity, and guilt.

Not unlike the mythical three-minute mile and the .500 batting average, locker room statistics ("How many times?" and "How often?") cause a deep chasm of fear felt in the bedroom.

Metathoughts like "I hope I can perform tonight," "I hope she gets aroused," "There's no fool like an old fool" crowd the water bed.

If we examine how we are changing, how we are caught between two contradictory points of view, how the locker-room game is but another fairy tale, and how our fears develop, then our performance might improve, and our "rolls in the hay" might become more who we really are in mid-life.

Sexual Conditioning of the 1940s and 1950s

Our sexual conditioning is premised on two contrary views. The first holds that *sex is manhood* and the second that *sex is bad.* Together these views placed early definitions of "Who am I?" in a precarious position.

The average male child grows up equating sex with competitiveness, being masterful, being responsible, direct, and forceful. Translated into Freudian slips, he learns to make it, to be on top, to come together, and to have a big one.

This superstandard view is continued into adolescence. Our sexual dreams on library days became so strong many of us grew up thinking the Dewey Decimal System was another name for the rhythm method. From our localized growing pains in junior high, we moved to our first score, a time when talking about it afterward seemed more important than the act itself. Remember how smug you were the next day in homeroom? This newfound power was constantly reinforced by the football players and rock stars. Take Tom, for example. Tom is a forty-six-year-old, good-looking supersalesman who became a member of a middle-aged men's counseling group. Notice how he epitomizes the Stud U.S.A. point of view.

Tom: I have this recurring dream to screw women I see during the day. Just once, mind you ... but I'd love to do that.

Jerry (a fellow group member): Only once ... why not more?

Tom: No ... just once.

Jerry: I still don't understand why you would only want them once if they were good.

Tom: Hey, I don't know! I guess I don't want to get involved.

Jerry: Then what you are saying is that you don't want a woman too close to you.

Tom: I don't know! I just want to screw them ... that's all ... just once.

This forties and fifties conditioning about manliness is but a remnant in the conscious minds of most of us, as it is in Tom's. Yet it is the conditioning that continues into adult life and leaves us half in and half out of bed.

The second point of view held that sex is bad—something only for dirty old men. A careful look at the forties and fifties indicates it was based on a man's taking advantage of a sweet young thing. We were guilty. Tony, a 45-year-old appliance salesman, is still having trouble with this:

Tony: I met this beautiful girl on a trip to Texas. One thing led to another and I took her to bed. It was great, but the next morning I could hardly look at her. I really took advantage of her.

Larry (a fellow group member, asking Tony why he felt guilty): She was 18 years old and able to vote.

Tony: Yeah, but if I hadn't pushed it—well, you know—the after-dinner drinks. I guess I could forget it except now when I make love to my wife I get impotent right in the middle of it. I can't seem to help it. I keep thinking about that night in Texas.

We are, then, products of a schizophrenic existence—caught between two points of view. One voice whispers that we are the aggressor and should get all we can, and the other tells us if we do we'll feel guilty for taking advantage of that sweet young thing.

Masters and Johnson comment on this vestige of Victorianism:

The cultural concept of the male partner who must accept full responsibility of establishing successful coital connection has placed upon every man a psychological burden for the coital process and has released every woman from any suggestion of semi-responsibility for a success.[1]

Sexual Hang-Ups

What are the sexual hang-ups that affect The Gray Itch? Generally these are (a) a residual sense of guilt; (b) male separation of sex from love; (c) sex equated with manhood; (d) female body worship; (e) spectator point of view; (f) separation of sex from work, and (g) the longing to be a sexual twenty-year-old.

In days of old when men were bold, we were allowed to think of sex as fun—but as an act, performed only with guilt. For years we lived with a hang-up brought about by the feeling in our pants and the amount of guilt in our heads. Our culture stressed action, responsibility, positiveness on the part of the male, and offered few opportunities for getting any. An interesting dichotomy. Remember those encounters in the Chevy or Ford? Myron Brenton explains in *The American Male:* "In those days, the boys tried to get all they could and the girl put her budding femininity to work to keep his sexual interest high, but his sexual accomplishments low.[2]

By mid-life, then, most of us have built up an excessive number of "guilties" related to the division between sexual thoughts and actions. Unfortunately, this residual sense of guilt often affects the sexual self-esteem of the middle-aged man to the point where he is confused about who he is and, thus, what he should be in bed.

The separation of sex and love often is an unwanted hang-up in the middle-aged man's search for continuing sexual identity. While he has been conditioned to this separation, his basic need in mid-life may be a reaffirmation of his total self, love, and intimacy. Thanks to our contrary points of view, we often find ourselves estranged from the thing we need the most, a loving relationship. Jim reinforces this point:

I like sex as well as the next guy, but now I also want to walk in a sunset with a woman or take a bath with her. Every time I take a girl out now it's like a sexual trial run at Indianapolis. I really enjoy a quiet evening just watching TV or holding a woman, not just competing for the rail position.

Another hang-up with a paradoxical twist is seen in the middle-aged man who is unable to separate sex from manhood. If this person fails sexually, he fails as a man! Deep and continuing sexual references to "making it" have been woven into the fabric of our lives, cowboy boots, and machismo. Only a man makes a woman.

An additional hang-up of the forties and fifties is female body worship. From watching Sally's panties on the playground bars in kindergarten to sitting baldheaded in the front row of the Moulin Rouge Burlesque in old age, men tend to objectify women into a nicely turned leg, a hip, or a breast. From overt statements like "Look at that one" to a subtle elbow from one male teenager to another on the beach, the cultural conditioning is reinforced. Into mid-life the sex-object worship becomes private mutterings and a deep breath, followed by an empty feeling in the groin, as we watch the file girl walk down the hall in front of us.

Ironically we become physically less in body than we were, yet we step up our looking at the female body. We buy one-way mirrored sunglasses, spend more time at the beach, and watch pornos as we stand before the urinal in Ripple's Restaurant in San Francisco.

There are several reasons for body-worship fantasy. Our cultural conditioning condones body worship, but only vicariously. Our wives tell us it's all right to look but not touch; female streakers actually run unmolested through crowds of hard hats. To look and not touch presumes the objects are like mannequins in a store window, desired but possessing little soul or personality. Thus, for some males our spectator-voyeur appreciation reduces women to mere objects.

This sort of spectator conditioning is continually reinforced by television ads that sell autos with breasts that hang out over the car door, and girls on bicycles with undersized seats. The viewer can only act forceful if he buys toothpaste, a new car, or a bicycle.

Small wonder that in mid-life one finds himself emasculated as a viewmaster, a voyeur, conditioned to look and not touch. Occasionally, as a result, he detaches himself and becomes a spectator in a sexual relationship. He drops out during the act, to watch his partner and himself. He remains in the bleacher seats during the game. To him the mirrors and the bathroom light become more important than the touch. But what does this do to the side of him that demands action? Part of the problem of secondary impotence in middle age is related to the fact that we become spectators. In relation to the spectator role, Masters and Johnson state:

Dysfunctional people have become so fearful of their own performance that they mentally watch themselves and their reactions during sexual activity instead of just allowing the natural feeling to take over.[3]

Old 1940s and 1950s hang-ups have also cut and torn our sex lives from our work. This does not mean that many serious affairs aren't initiated around the water cooler or that "sticking your pen in the company ink" isn't still an important sport within the corporation. But the overriding Puritan ethic offers work as primary and sexual activity as secondary. For years we have, because of the "competition" or striving to be a company man, sublimated our sex lives to almighty work. "For the good of the company," we have worked our butts off, while finding time for getting some becomes a matter of chance at home. The work ethic allowed sex to literally and figuratively take a back seat.

A further hang-up that is put on the metapausal man is that the Victorian double standard no longer exists. Today we find young ladies—and some not so young—who talk about their sexual experience like a sports announcer, who go to bed to see if they like you, who masturbate, who don't want children, who take the Pill, and who assume the upper position without asking. Coupled with newer concepts of neuter sexuality, it's difficult for the middle-aged man to adjust to changing standards.

Our Victorian backgrounds have dicated abstinence (which we never followed, right?). Today the new ethic seems to imply that we should try to "wear it out." How about communal life, singles apartments, and touchie-feelie groups? The swinger ethic seems to have few guilties, no regrets, no hangups, and fewer pregnancies. Look at what we missed! Wouldn't it be wonderful to be twenty again! A certain sense of sexual nostalgia creeps over many of us; we feel we've been cheated, and The Gray Itch increases.

We are indeed the products of a time and place, with two points of view about sex. We are metapausal men who wonder about our sexual preoccupations, feel guilt yet desire, fear yet responsibility, and all the while are constantly infused with the thought of how we are physically changing.

By the Numbers

Probably foremost in the sexual conditioning of the middle-aged man are the myths that surrounded "doing it by the numbers." Remember the locker-room bragging? How about those friends of your big brother's who used to boast . . . "we screwed five or six times during intermission in the drive-in." As we get older, the exaggerations are fewer, but the numbers game still remains an important part of our sexuality. We might only have had a "C" average in math, but we all need to be "A" students in the mythical game of sexual powers. Unfortunately, in mid-life we continue to take these numbers games to bed with us. It's easy to see that our sexual prestige oneupmanship, if you will, is often expressed in terms of numbers in a society that puts a premium on quantity rather than quality. It isn't surprising that to prove who we are sexually, inches, times per week, or the number of orgasms become quite important.

Length-of-Penis Myth. From the Greek urn paintings to Breughel's hay-gathering scenes to *Deep Throat*, myths about the size of the penis are legend. Well, how long is the average penis in the flaccid state? Masters and Johnson found that, of the men in their study, the smallest penis in the flaccid state measured just under two and a half inches, while the largest was five and a half inches long.

Size-of-Erection Myth. The next myth came into our minds the first time we entered the shower room in junior high. This myth relates to the comparative size of the male penis in a flaccid state as compared to a fully erected one. Masters and Johnson again attest that "the soft penis does vary in size from individual to individual but this variation is much less during erection." The average erect penis is 6 inches, with most men varying between four and a half to eight inches. Masters and Johnson further found that smaller penises doubled in size at the height of sexual excitement, while larger penises generally did not increase much.

The How-Often Myth. Another quantity myth should also bite the dust. This myth has it that some men do it all the time; they rock around the clock. "How many times did you get her?" asks a twenty-year-old of his friend. "Oh, about six or seven, I think—I forget." "In two hours?" asks the first. The number of times the average married couple has sexual intercourse is somewhere around one to three times a week. One researcher found that men in their 40's have sex an average of one and a half times a week.[4]

The Number of Orgasms Myth. The next myth relates to the slide rule of the American sexual encounter—the number of orgasms. There is a great similarity between the sexes, but the sexual-response cycle of each is quite different. After completing the orgasm, the male needs a longer period before another orgasm is possible. In younger men this period is shorter (about 10 minutes) and longer in middle-aged men (at least a half hour for another erection). The female can remain at sexual tension. Over 50 percent of females are capable of several orgasms in minutes according to Masters and Johnson.[5] The main reason this occurs is that the female erective chambers refill with blood immediately after orgasm and create a new sexual tension.

The Simultaneous-Orgasm Myth. Another myth relates to the colossal technical feat of simultaneous orgasm. To expect an instantaneous orgasm each time is like preparing for D-day in bed. "Making the effort to coordinate such basically involuntary responses starts partners observing themselves mentally, rather than losing themselves in the feeling of love-making."[6]

The Four-Hour Intercourse Myth. This expectation relates to the numbers games of "We screwed for hours and hours and tore down trees, shrubs, and flowers." These barroom exaggerations are worldwide and not only run counter to limited evidence but put more pressure on the middle-aged man's performance as well.

The Orgasm Myth. Still another is the size of the orgasm. Those who boast that they have had a large orgasm trace it to the fact that they emitted a great deal of semen during ejaculation. This barroom baloney has little basis in fact. Evidence indicates that about the same amount of semen is ejaculated by all of us, although the strength of the psychological orgasm can be more at times than at others. Unquestionably, the evidence indicates that the magnitude of the orgasm is psychological and not related to the quantity of semen ejaculated.

First Fears

In mid-life first fears of sexual adequacy can become fears of losing who we are. As a friend once said, "From the twenties to the forties, I walked around as if I had racing stripes on my penis. When I got to the forties, my racing days were over."

As we have seen, some of the "who-am-I" concept of the American male is carried between his legs. Then, in mid-life, the guys in the bar start telling jokes about "not keeping it up," and the wife brings home a joke from the bridge table: "What are the three two-letter words that can destroy a man?" Answer: "Is it in?" A cold chill goes down his back. Jokes like these make many of us feel as if we should turn in our track suits. If we can't run a three-minute mile, last an hour in the saddle, or pole-vault into bed every night, we become fearful.

Unfortunately, numbers-game fears cause the middle-aged man problems in sexual performance. We find we are unable to meet these mythical standards (quantifications of so many, so fast, and so big). Just as we were unable to pull ourselves up to peep into our neighbor's bedroom window at age ten, so is the middle-aged man unable to separate his sexual myths from realities.

Before we examine some of the specific first fears of sexual metapause, there's something that should be understood. With normal aging and halfway decent health, a man can have an active sex life well past his retirement. Again, Masters and Johnson point out: "A man in good health who has a partner in whom he is interested should enjoy an active sex life even in his eighties." [7] Now, that makes you feel better, doesn't it?

After that reassurance let's look at some of the sexual changes in us.

Sexual Arousal Time. One of the initial sexual fears that a middle-aged man has is that it seems to take him a longer time to become aroused. The excitement phase usually takes more time for the middle-aged man. It takes longer to get an erection, and the erection may not be as hard initially as when he was younger. Unfortunately, many of us jump into bed as they do in a five-minute porno and expect the thing in our hands to understand. It doesn't. Our lack of understanding of the aging process causes us to become at least frustrated, and at worst scared to death. Losing an erection is like being fired.

Semen Reduction. Another physical change that occurs in us is that we do not ejaculate the same amount of semen as we grow older. Expulsion of semen is less forceful in older men and there is not as much seminal fluid as in younger men.

Again, we begin to worry about those first fears ("I wonder what she thinks." "I bet others don't have these problems"). We can't get much help from our cronies, either, for they are still bragging about their four-hour rides, even though most of it is oneupmanship. Masters and Johnson found that the reduction of semen is noticeable as we age. Most of us who discharge less fluid feel that, indeed, we have lost our racing stripes, and some tend to blame their partners for their lack of stimulation. The average middle-aged man doesn't seem to understand that ejaculation is an important aspect of orgasm, but the amount of semen is but a mythical quantification of his orgasm.

Psychological Frequency of Sex. Another sexual problem within The Gray Itch is that the number of sexual encounters per week does reduce as we and our marriage age. You can't do as many push-ups as you once did, right? The problem is the same, even though it may be more psychological than physical. If first fears exist in the middle-aged man's mind, or if the wife feels, "That's for the younger folks," or they watch "The Tonight Show" diligently, or she thinks of how much the bedroom ceiling needs painting, the problem may not be physical at all. It may be purely psychological—the need for new motivation, interest, excitement. Take Ruth's comment to a counselor concerning this problem, after considerable discussion between them.

Counselor: How is your sex life, Ruth?
Ruth: Well, I think it's good, Ben [her husband] never complained. He seems happy. Of course, we don't make love very often anymore.... You know, when you get older you don't, do you?

In Ruth's comments we see a part of conventional wisdom that gives poor Ben the feeling his next one may be his last one.

Research on the subject indicates there is a declining frequency of sexual relations in mid-life. But this declining frequency may be directly related to changes that are psychological instead of physical. One counselee said:

In 20 years ... yeah, 20 years, once we made love on the couch in front of the T.V. and once in the shower. I get tired of putting the dog out and of the Missionary position with the lights out.

The Orgasm Compulsion. First fears are also encountered when the middle-aged man finds that his overwhelming need to have an orgasm during sexual intercourse seems to lessen. He then wonders if it's him or his partner. Yet many are probably able to satisfy their partner better now with "delayed reaction" than when they were a compulsive eighteen.

Women also change as they grow older, and their changing reactions affect our ability to perform and produce additional fears in us.

Arousal for a female also takes longer as she ages. Many men feel that something is lacking in their technique or in female interest when middle-aged women take longer to become aroused than younger women. During sexual arousal time the average female's vaginal lubrication occurs somewhat more slowly, and less lubricant is produced as she grows older. Younger women take fifteen to thirty seconds to become lubricated, while it may take one to three minutes of sex play to initiate it in older women. This fact confuses many middle-aged men, who assume that their faulty technique or poor performance is responsible for slower arousal.[8]

Moreover, women seem to respond more to the total person and the total situation as they get older. Thus, men want the light on, women want it off; women want to be loved, men wish to be satisfied. The reaction in each is dependent upon the significant differences in early sexual conditioning which become exaggerated in mid-life.

Without understanding these and other kinds of sexual changes that occur within us, many metapausal men in middle age become fearful of who they are and often become subject to two main sexual problems: secondary impotence and premature ejaculation.

However, most of our problems about sexual performance are in our heads. Masters and Johnson state: "The susceptibility of the human male to the power of suggestion with regard to his sexual prowess is almost . . . unbelievable." [9]

Secondary Impotence. At the center of secondary impotence are many of our fears. Sooner or later, in some sexual encounter, secondary impotence occurs in all of us. During an unsuccessful encounter, fear turns into panic. Our minds and our penises seem to question each other, become uncoordinated, or lack a basic understanding. Very often, secondary impotence is related to several important factors in the middle-aged man. He tries to force himself to get ready, forgetting that his two-minute warmup days are over. And then there is alcohol. Masters and Johnson found excessive alcohol consumption to be a primary characteristic of secondary impotence. While there is no conclusive scientific evidence on the subject, some evidence shows that if a middle-aged man has fears of sexual inadequacy, he keeps fortifying himself with French Beaujolais long after his partner is ready for a French kiss.

Probably one of the greatest causes of secondary impotence is the anxiety produced when metathoughts such as "maybe I can't satisfy her" or "I want to last through her orgasm" enter our heads.

Hormone Loss. Hormone output, particularly of testosterone, does decline in mid-life, and after. The decline is usually gradual, with the greatest drop between ages forty and fifty.[10] Only 10 to 15 percent of males suffer from an abrupt decline, however. The good news is that potency is not related to how much hormones is stimulated by our pituitary at any one time. The bad news is that a gradual loss does affect our interest in sex. But by age seventy, the sperm count is about a third of what it was at age thirty-five.[11] Although he may take longer to get aroused and ejaculate, with good health and an amenable partner, a man should be able to function sexually until he dies of old age.

Premature Ejaculation. Premature ejaculation is the second occurrence that panics many middle-aged men. As we have seen, our conditioning of the forties and fifties has given the total responsibility for the sexual act to the male. As the sexual controller, the responsible one, men find themselves in the position of directing the entire production. As a director, males abstract themselves from deep involvement in the process so that they can make sure that their partner is satisfied and that the conditions of their performance contract are met. This dropping out or abstracting seems to cause the observer to become a spectator, a symptom related to erective failure or premature ejaculation. Once again, expert opinion is given by Masters and Johnson:

Man deliberately blocks off sexually stimulating signals from his wife instead of losing himself in the natural response of her caresses, her bodily movement, her facial expression. He abstracts himself from these and concentrates only on avoiding ejaculation. Over a period of years, this deliberate blocking of sexual stimuli leads to an episode of erective failure. In the case of premature ejaculation, the problem of failing as a man is not physically reacting, but his failure to satisfy his wife or lover. The female role becomes crucial in the whole area of premature ejaculation. A number of mental distractions such as counting backwards from a hundred and thinking of a business problem or a recalling of a vacation trip are certain strategies that have been used by men in the past. But these techniques fail because they tend to distract from the love relationship which in turn can lead to some secondary impotency problems.[12]

From kindergarten to mid-life, then, we are conditioned to judge who we are sexually. Sexual identity and The Gray Itch are translated into a numbers game that few in early life and only a handful in mid-life can win. As we grow older, we are still able to prove who we are sexually, but only after the mythology is examined and classified for what it is. We can do it and get Social Security, too, but most of us fear we're about to lose it because we are unaware of the exaggerated mythology and the fact that we are changing.

H.I.M.M.
(Hallberg Index of Male Metapause)

SEXUAL I.D.

The statements that follows represent some of your present and future feelings and concerns about metapause in the area of your sex life.

DIRECTIONS

Please mark each statement twice. First, mark with a circle one number for each statement to represent your nearest current feeling about the subject. Second, mark one number with a square to represent where you wish to see yourself regarding the statement. Higher numbers should equal stronger feelings.

EXAMPLE

I enjoy taking the
initiative in lovemaking.   1   2   3   ④   5   6   7   8̄   9   10

SEX CONTINUUM

1. I enjoy taking the in-   1   2   3   4   5   6   7   8   9   10
   itiative in love-
   making

2. Sometimes I feel   1   2   3   4   5   6   7   8   9   10
   like a spectator
   while making love.

3. I'm so tired when I   1   2   3   4   5   6   7   8   9   10
   get home from work
   that I rarely feel like
   sex.

4. I sometimes have   1   2   3   4   5   6   7   8   9   10
   questions about the
   size of my penis.

5. I can't seem to get an   1   2   3   4   5   6   7   8   9   10
   erection as fast as I
   once did.

6. I have real fears   1   2   3   4   5   6   7   8   9   10
   about impotence.

7. My wife doesn't   1   2   3   4   5   6   7   8   9   10
   seem to be inter-
   ested in sex.

8. After sex I fall asleep immediately.

    1 2 3 4 5 6 7 8 9 10

9. I wish my wife and I could have an orgasm together.

    1 2 3 4 5 6 7 8 9 10

10. I satisfy her sexually.

    1 2 3 4 5 6 7 8 9 10

11. I lose my potency sometimes in the middle of the sex act.

    1 2 3 4 5 6 7 8 9 10

12. My wife/girl friend seems to warm up more slowly these days.

    1 2 3 4 5 6 7 8 9 10

13. I'm not interested in sex with my wife.

    1 2 3 4 5 6 7 8 9 10

14. I think my wife and I have sex fewer times a month than the average.

    1 2 3 4 5 6 7 8 9 10

15. I feel that I need to be the director in the sex act.

    1 2 3 4 5 6 7 8 9 10

16. I would like to have sex with a different woman every day.

    1 2 3 4 5 6 7 8 9 10

17. I wish I could have sexual experiences more frequently.

    1 2 3 4 5 6 7 8 9 10

18. I masturbate quite often.   1 2 3 4 5 6 7 8 9 10

19. I feel that drinking before making love makes me a better lover.   1 2 3 4 5 6 7 8 9 10

20. I like big-breasted women.   1 2 3 4 5 6 7 8 9 10

SCORING

Now add up the sum total of your circled numbers and your squared numbers and enter them below:

○ Circled Score: _____   □ Squared Score: _____

A comparison of your scores can be obtained in two steps:

1. Compare your own current and wished for scores on each statement.
2. If a difference of more than twenty points exists between your *total* current and wished for scores, refer to the corresponding Metacare Guidelines in Chapter 12.

Chapter 7

FOR BETTER OR
FOR WORSE

Even the natural expression of "Who am I?" in the young and developing marriage gets buried under bills and bicycles, doesn't it? The middle-aged man, once cast as a protector and known as a "good provider" through his silver anniversary, suddenly finds his wife needs to get away for a few days. As the last word in the family authority system, he has trouble getting a word in edgewise and finds everybody is doing his "own thing."

One morning, as his struggle for "Who am I?" reaches deep down into the cup of black instant coffee he made, his mutterings become audible through munches on his instant breakfast-food bar: "What happened to our marriage?" "For better or worse, that's ridiculous." "For richer or poorer, what does that mean?" These are new metathoughts about yet another area of "Who am I?" for the metapausal man.

Well, what did happen? What happened to the double standard, Doris Day, and "A Sleepy Lagoon"? What happened to "the missus," as you used to call her? Where's the romance? Just what happened?

We know through studies that the satisfaction often goes out of marriage in mid-life. In a *Family* magazine study of U.S. marriages, very few reported qualitatively good marriages. In another study the smallest percentage of marital satisfaction appeared in mid-life—before the launching and postparental periods of child rearing—with sixty-six percent of the husbands feeling less than satisfied and only 9–24 percent very satisfied with their marriages.[1] By the way, middle-aged wives felt the same. Another study reported only 6 percent of the wives said they were fully satisfied with marriage after 20 or more years.[2]

That middle-aged marriages are in trouble today is further confirmed by a U.S. Bureau of the Census study that shows the highest incidence of divorce and separation for men is between the ages of 40 and 44, excluding the initial adjustment period. Divorce seems to be on the increase. In 1974 there were 2,223,000 marriages in the U.S. and 970,000 divorces.

It appears that our personal questions about marriage in mid-life are not merely our own; statistics bear out that many others feel the same.

Let's see what marriage means to old Lester who recently underwent group counseling:

I walked around, thinking how nice it would be to be free of marriage, of this house. But, I can't leave the kids. They need me and, really, my life isn't so bad. Elaine keeps a fairly clean house, and she certainly spends an inordinate amount of time keeping the children clean. And, now that I'm less interested in work as in previous times, I should be more involved with the family. But, it isn't very important to me. We all seem to be bored. We get up at the same time, do the same things, even what we eat each week seems predictable. What's our purpose in life? What are we married for now?

Within Lester's statement we can clearly see shifts in his metathoughts about his wife and kids, his feelings about freedom and responsibility, and his feelings about himself.

Lester's statement today is quite different from what he said as he raised his glass of Chianti before his bride-to-be twenty-five years ago. He dedicated himself as a provider, welded himself into a lifetime partnership, indentured himself by choice to protect his betrothed, and fantasized to himself about the next night's activity, which would eventually lead him to a greater purpose—a son, also named Lester. Knowing the rough road ahead, his middle-aged in-laws, aunts, and uncles sat around the checkered tablecloth smiling approvingly, smiling as though they had just eaten a hot pepper and needed to say "Excuse me."

Today, Lester feels knee-deep in the sands of easy credit, climbing up yet one more hill. Further trapped in his commitment to the institution of marriage with a changing or unknown purpose, Lester would like his enlistment canceled.

We see in marriage as in other areas of "Who am I?" that our identity changes because our marriage changes. Our marriage identity has three basic aspects: one, how we look at ourselves in marriage; two, how our partners look at us; and three, how strong is our sense of purpose to remain married.

Inside, how does Lester look at his marriage?

First, in the past, his inside marriage identity developed through "macho-me" roles that told him that his wife changed the diapers and had the dinner on the table. He washed the car and screwed things into the wall, shouted, and drank straight whiskey. Today all he sees in the mirror is the family accountant, Sally's husband, or a man named Daddy. These fixed roles leave little room for him in mid-life.

Lester's marriage identity is reflected outside by his wife. In mid-life she, too, has problems. She wants to be free after dedicating her adult life to raising the kids. She wants to set out to accomplish some of her own goals instead of feeding off the ambitions of her husband or the kids. Striking out for a job or the local university, she takes long strides in her own direction. And Lester is left wondering what's going on as his marriage changes further.

At the very time when making it at work seems less important to him, Lester's wife begins to turn left at Oak Street each morning. Confused by these changes, his sense of self is continually buffeted by the winds of his disengagement from his marriage.

With fixed roles inside and a changing partner outside, the identity developed through his marriage becomes difficult to decode in mid-life.

We must also examine what happens in mid-life to the purposes for marriage, the third and possibly most important part of the metapausal marriage identity puzzle. The "P" in purpose for marriage can be defined by six other "P's": partnership, procreation, protection, provision, penetration, and propinquity. These words define Lester's purpose and represent 99 percent of the toasts at Mario's twenty-five years ago. Let's look at each and see if it is still a part of our purpose for marriage in mid-life.

"Marriage is a Partnership"

"I now join you as man and wife," "Two can live as cheaply as one," "Two heads are better than one." A partnership is formed—in sales, in production, in administration, in stores, and in accounting.

As with the struggle for the other five "P's," the purpose of partnership demands two shoulders to the wheel. Thelma C. Purtell said:

We often call marriage a closed corporation. A corporation is a business venture; so is marriage. What with filling out forms jointly and each exemption carefully noted, with budgets and buying and acquiring real estate and investing in the future—stocks for retirement, education for the children—it is Big Business.[5]

What happens in mid-life when the struggle becomes less, overcome by previous accomplishments? What happens when the wheel becomes greased? What happens when there seems to be less competition or struggle for a successful partnership? In a way, what happens when we have it made? If we have joined in a partnership to overcome obstacles and accomplish other purposes such as protection, providing, and procreating, what happens to the partnership when the other purposes are no longer important? Do we dissolve the partnership, declare bankruptcy?

Ironically, once having "made it," much of the "infighting" within the marriage corporation continues to be over the legal tender of the partnership—money. Nearly 40 percent of all troubles of husbands and wives who reach forty develop around money; either the lack of it or the management of it.[6]

"Think of the Children"

So let's look for purpose in the second "P," procreation. Certainly today, the way you and your wife look at each other over breakfast when she is five days overdue settles that one. Procreation is hardly a main reason anymore, is it? If you have any doubts, try to remember the last time your wife subtly said, "John, did you know that Harry got a vasectomy and Sarah said that he said it didn't hurt a bit?"

But there is more to producing children. We need to raise them. Yet even this reason for marriage seems to be fading. Larry finishes law school next year, and Jenny is living with the "family" on a commune somewhere in Arizona.

Returning home early one evening, David, an assembly-line foreman, said to his wife, "I bought a pool table today for Gloria's old room." Or, "I'm going to take the lock off our bedroom door, okay?" Each is an indication that the marriage purpose of procreation is a thing of the past in David's mind.

The need to parent goes far beyond begetting and raising children, for soon there may be grandchildren. But is this sufficient justification to continue the marriage contract, an important metathought of the metapausal man.

"I'm the Breadwinner"

Providing is the next part of purpose. You really thought you had a corner on this one until recently, didn't you? Now, joint expense accounts and separate income tax schedules take the fun out of it. Instead of carrying in a stag on your shoulder and throwing it down on the table amid accolades from the family, your wife makes more than you do and she asks you one night what would happen if she got transferred to Cleveland?

Providing is a particularly difficult issue for the middle-aged man who is identified so closely with his work. His outward expression of his work value is often that 10 percent raise or stock option. If his wife's plan offers great annuities, free dental and psychological and medical care, and use of the company jet, how significant does his bow and arrow remain?

What happens to the hunter who no longer hunts? What happens to his manhood, inseparably woven into the fabric of his work? What happens to the hunter when the "little woman's" work calls her away or she calls and tells him she is going to lay over in Cincinnati because of a snowstorm?

Mixing feelings of entrapment in the business enterprises and at home on the one hand, and his need for freedom on the other, the middle-aged man becomes a prime target of The Gray Itch. Yet any man who doesn't meet his responsibilities—braces, house payments, college tuition—clearly isn't a man. Generally translated into dollars and cents, male responsibility for "providing"—a thirty-year marriage, eight years of college—forms a long-term lien on his person, a person who may wish to escape to freedom. Instead, he feels he is on a forced march, plodding through a jungle of responsibilities

"Who Needs Protection"

Examination of the next part of purpose for marriage—protection—isn't much help, either. Conditioned into the average American male is the expectation that he will protect the weaker sex partner he married. "Didn't I protect the whole damn world during the *war?*" he laments. "Look at all those hash marks, and that fruit salad." Was there any doubt when you returned after five years in the Pacific to the girl next door that you were to be her protector? In those days women still took the inside position on the sidewalk and liked it. Until recently, the fragile girl didn't play football, ride as a jockey, or even go into a bar alone. Now it's "Anything you can do, I can do better."

Most disconcerting to you, however, is not that you aren't asked to protect the wife and kids, but deep down—don't tell anybody—you wonder if you still can. "Yes, but I was in the boxing team in college," you counter. Fine, but how many muggers, rapists, and robbers are overcome by middle-aged boxers? And anyway, how can a twenty-year-old lightweight box at fifty, as a heavyweight? After a night of the six o'clock news and "Policewoman," you really aren't sure, are you?

One day your eighteen-year-old daughter comes chopping through the front door and announces she's a black belt in karate and proceeds to show you her progress. As you look up at her from the floor, clutching at your old war injury, you wonder further about your protective powers.

Of the first four original purposes for marriage, then, we have zero for four in mid-life. Partnership, procreation, providing, and protection seem to be questionable reasons for continuing the enterprise of marriage. Is it any wonder another mirror of who you are becomes foggy in mid-life?

As you may recall, we set out to see how male metapause was affected by marriage. We discussed the middle-aged man's feelings of entrapment related to his inside and outside identity and some aspects of the continuing purposes for his marriage. Penetration is yet another part of purpose, the fifth.

From the early sexual experience to the middle-aged man's alleged sexual decline, male psychology plays an important part in sexuality.

Remember when you were eighteen, desiring release, sitting night after night in the 1952 Ford in front of her house? Night after night, you played it "cool" or you were aggressive, wrestling, even cajoling, but to no avail. You greatest release was when you finally unsnapped her bra, on the seventh date.

In mid-life the metapausal man's physical ability probably doesn't decline half as fast as his psychological ability to get turned on. Reciting the alphabet in the same order night after night for twenty years cancels anticipation. The ritual of (a) taking a bath, (b) putting out the dog, (c) using your hand warmer, (d) locking the door, (e) pulling the drapes, (f) turning the radio low becomes a computerized countdown and blocks the participants from intimacy.

Penetration seems to lack the excitement, the chase, hunt, and submission. Look at the jokes that condition us for psychological changes in bed. From early adulthood's "We screwed for hours and hours," to mid-life's "It takes all night to do what I used to do all night!"

One study reports that by the age fifty, 49 percent of the men and 58 percent of the women admitted to some decline in their sexual interest and activity, with the sharpest increase of this awareness occurring between the ages of forty-five and fifty-five.[7]

One bored lover wrote, "You can only seduce your wife once." Unfortunately, few middle-aged men consciously recognize that they are psychologically not with it in bed.

Another part of the psychological problem related to the continuing purpose of marriage involves the subtle changes that occur in his and in her sexual expectations. In mid-life, she may feel safer, have what Masters and Johnson call "freedom from fear" and have a tendency to get more turned on. In these cases, the middle-aged woman decides that procreation was really only an excuse to learn how to do it, and now she becomes much more aggressive. The middle-aged man sometimes is unable to cope with this shift in attitude.

Other women in their forties and preparing early for Social Security feel sex in mid-life is like drinking beer—once or twice a year at most.

Whichever of these positions the middle-aged woman takes, it makes the bedroom a different place for the middle-aged man. Even with the development of new techniques, *More Joy of Sex,* and new liberation for women, penetration can hardly be the reason for keeping "Mr. and Mrs." on the mailbox. Let's look at the last purpose for continuing this 25-year marriage—propinquity.

Now we face a very illusive word meaning closeness, intimacy, love, and caring. You middle-aged males would say that's "women stuff." Well, maybe. However, most psychologists believe we all need some types of intimacy, some strokes, what the transactional analysts call "warm fuzzies." The need for emotional support and intimacy develops in all human beings, male and female, at a very young age. Babies die if not touched physically or attended to throughout early life. One often develops a negative self-image if unloved or uncared for by others.

In mid-life, the need for warmth, tenderness, trust, and a hug may become even more important. Do you realize there may may be a linear yearly decline in the number of times partners kiss from that first toast at Mario's to mid-life? Loss of intimate interaction involving kissing, confiding, and reciprocity has been found to be the second largest factor contributing to marital disenchantment in mid-life.[8]

A lack of "agreement between partners about affection" contributes mostly to this loss of intimate interaction. Listen to what Jack, 47, told his group:

I'm really confused sometimes. I mean, I live in a house full of people and I'm lonely. I really can't talk to anyone about the things that bother me, least of all my wife. I need her to care now more than ever and she doesn't seem to understand that. She's almost patronizing.

Jack not only wants intimacy, but needs it. And if he doesn't get it, his emptiness might lead to ways of "acting out" his need. In *The American Male* we learn:

As for married men of 35 or so, the ones who have a number of years of marriage behind them, should an early, romantic bloom wither, their feelings of matrimony, as a manner of greater benefit to women more than men, well may intensify. If this happens, the feeling of being trapped grows stronger. The result, not infrequently, is alcoholism, infidelity, or both—and, finally, divorce.[9]

We have established that the need for propinquity exists, that all of us need care and feeding of our intimate needs.

If everybody needs intimacy, why isn't it more a part of the marriage scene? We practice the piano, law, medicine, and golf. Why don't we practice intimacy? Why, if it's so important to keep the middle-aged man buying anniversary presents, don't we practice being intimate?

The family enterprise, adapting to constant pressures during its first twenty-five years, is basically a business enterprise with a few "fringes." As a green-eyeshade accountant, banker, laborer, carpenter, TV repairman, you struggled to make an investment in marriage. You struggled to reach new family benchmarks—a new car, a house, a college education for your children. How often has your wife said, "Don't you feel we should buy a new sofa, Harry?" Or, "The car is going to need new tires and transmission work. How about a Porsche?" you ask her. It's the American way, isn't it?

You and your wife feed the "move-up" syndrome, shoving bonus checks, income tax refunds, and raises into the boiler that generates more need to buy—at the expense of your propinquity. It doesn't make much sense, does it, to put that two-hundred-dollar leather jacket around your emptiness?

If, in fact, intimacy or propinquity is the last surviving "P" in marriage, it will have difficult sledding. If this single survivor of purpose is slipped between locking the front door, driving the kids to school, or buying a new sofa, then no wonder the middle-aged man questions his marriage. If this closeness is so important, then every day must be like Father's Day and Mother's Day. Generally, each day isn't.

Confused and unsure of himself, the metapausal man begins a process of "acting out" The Gray Itch. Unknowingly, he blames his marriage partner or himself, laying out a sophisticated rationale. Or he buys a truckload of bricks and proceeds to build a wall around himself, disengaging himself from the marriage while remaining at home. These stick-to-it types, for the sake of the neighbors, boss, church, or the kids, remain "vowed" but not really wowed!

Then, of course, others look for another partner—at first just for a little excitement, "someone to talk to"—and an affair is spawned. More often today, separation and divorce are the solution to the Gray Itch. In his confusion the middle-aged man tries to find another mirror to reflect who he is.

Marital Disengagement

There is a calculable set of expectations for engagement in our society, and for disengagement from marriage as well. It appears all of these ways out of a marriage are based on a single principle of disengagement.

Sociological disengagement from activities and interpersonal involvement has long been claimed to be a process of aging.

For many the overt signs of disengagement that appear in

mid-life occur much later than actual disengagement. The reasons for this disengagement aren't difficult to figure out. Early division of responsibility, the child-rearing responsibilities of the wife and the corporate responsibilities of the husband, get the wheels rolling. Add to the recipe twenty years of having difficulty getting a word in sideways in a family conversation, add a pinch of conflict between husband and wife, and it's time to drop out and disengagement occurs.

These disengagements cause a downward spiral of communication for the couple who find in mid-life they have nothing to talk about. Old cartoons bear this out. Consider this one. The husband and wife are at the breakfast table, she in her robe and rollers, he in his matching robe and newspaper. She says, "George, I want a divorce." He says, "Yeah, it's going to be a hot one—probably up around 100°."

From the general concept of disengagement we must look at some typical ways middle-aged men "act out" marital dissatisfaction and their Gray Itch.

"It's Your Fault"

Modern-day psychology is filled with terms for the "it's-your-fault" syndrome: "The Prosecutor," "The Blamer," "If it weren't for you." Take Jim, for instance. He has some questions about himself, but in no way can he face them, so who gets it? The wife. It's her fault.

"The Poor Me"

The other side of the blamer or prosecutor way of "acting out" is "the poor me." This is often a call for sympathy. We feel depressed, we look at another 250 months of doing the bills, and we feel sorry for ourselves. We are victims! "Poor me" is a favorite of ours. Take Larry, bellied up at one of the local watering holes: "Oh, how I try. I buy her everything she wants, and what do I have to show for it? Nothing. I'm trapped." The best way to identify a "poor-me" victim is a series of catch phrases: "God, how I sacrificed for you." "Are you trying to make me crazy?" "Look how you have made me suffer." "If I treated you this way . . ." "What have I done to deserve this?" "How could you do this to me?" "It's her fault." "If only she didn't ..." "Why doesn't my wife understand me?"

All marriage relationships are nourished by an interaction between partners. Close times, mutual problems, and even friendly arguments are talked out; literally, related out in a communication network going two ways. Each "it's your fault" and "poor me" then is a complex but consistent expression of disengagement from marriage; the communication lines are cut. Either position isolates one from having to deal with the problem. If it is always the other person's problem, or if I feel sorry for myself, I get off the hook. Pain is translated into assumptions about the spouse. Because a two-way street is needed, complete communication is impossible. Assumptions are never tested but become "truisms" about the other partner, conjured up and empirically verified by their creator. A continuous script of blaming or self-pity develops, and disengagement continues.

Inside Dropout

Several other disengagements are typical of the metapausal man. The escape artist is one. With a sprinkling of hormonal change, late meetings, fixed roles, and some alcohol, the middle-aged man begins to mortar himself behind a wall at home. This disengaged but married character usually lives in but has dropped out. At the front door of the house he gives a casual "Hi" and retreats to his shop and model airplanes, his TV and beer, or his *Wall Street Journal* and classified ads.

One troubled woman told of a rash of family break ups in her neighborhood but proudly said of her husband, "Well, at least he's home." Holding on can be admirable, but seems hardly enough reason to continue marriage with an inside dropout.

Gauguin Syndrome

The reason we have the inside-dropout syndrome is that there's also the other side of the coin, an outside one. On a ski weekend at Lake Tahoe, one husband wrote his wife this postcard:

Hi. I'm having fun. Larry is fine and really having a ball in Tahoe.

He's changed his married look, taken off his ring and you should see the Danish doll he's dating ... her name is Karen, I think. She's only 22. I plan to stay another week.

There are season-pass ski tickets hanging around the wrinkled necks of middle-aged men. Suffering from the Gauguin syndrome, we find executives trading in their wingtips for bare feet in Florida; fathers in Alaska living alone, growing worms for the local fishermen; computer science experts cooking soufflés; and a middle-aged member of the ideal couple "just consulting" around while living on his 30-foot boat. All have The Gray Itch.

Stick-to-it-iveness

The stick-to-it-iveness type disengages from his marriage in a different way. He sticks with it because of the kids, boss, church, or neighbors, or so he thinks. Bill, a chain appliance-store manager, said:

I can't leave now. I might not make that promotion. There isn't a single head office director that isn't married. Besides, what would they say at the club. And, my kids would really reject me.

His outer pressures are an excuse for him to be miserable inside. At its extreme, he loses part of his stomach lining instead of leaving his wife.

We know the importance of parental modeling in raising children. Witness such syndromes as the battered child and alcoholism, which occur generation after generation. Kids, too, who often rarely see their stick-to-it-iveness fathers except when they are frothing at the mouth, are developing life scripts. Modeling, not heredity, is the prime factor. Modeling about love and marriage can be both positive and negative.

H.I.M.M.
(Hallberg Index of Male Metapause)

FOR BETTER OR WORSE

The statements that follow should represent some of your

present and future feelings and concerns about your marriage or living arrangements, as they relate to metapause.

DIRECTIONS

Please mark each statement twice. First, mark one number for each statement with a circle to represent your nearest current feeling about the subject. Second, mark one number with a square to represent where you wish to see yourself regarding the statement. Higher numbers should equal stronger feelings.

EXAMPLE

My wife and I aren't
close anymore.   1 ② 3 4 5 6 7 8̅ 9 10

FAMILY CONTINUUM

1. I work at home al-   1 2 3 4 5 6 7 8 9 10
   most every night.

2. I don't want any   1 2 3 4 5 6 7 8 9 10
   more control over
   family decisions.

3. I play an important   1 2 3 4 5 6 7 8 9 10
   role in my family to-
   day.

4. I'd retire right now 1 2 3 4 5 6 7 8 9 10
   and spend time with
   my wife if I could
   only afford it.

5. I don't have much   1 2 3 4 5 6 7 8 9 10
   hope for an exciting
   life and future in my
   marriage.

6. My home life is only a business.   1 2 3 4 5 6 7 8 9 10

7. If I had it to do over again, I wouldn't marry my wife.   1 2 3 4 5 6 7 8 9 10

8. I don't like my wife to get too close to me.   1 2 3 4 5 6 7 8 9 10

9. Who's got the time to be a loving person?   1 2 3 4 5 6 7 8 9 10

10. I tend to show my feelings to my wife.   1 2 3 4 5 6 7 8 9 10

11. I tend to talk a lot about my feelings.   1 2 3 4 5 6 7 8 9 10

12. When my wife is unreasonable, I usually keep my mouth shut and let her have her way.   1 2 3 4 5 6 7 8 9 10

13. I really get irritated these days at my wife over the smallest things.   1 2 3 4 5 6 7 8 9 10

14. I would never leave an unhappy marriage.   1 2 3 4 5 6 7 8 9 10

15. I always want to make more money than my wife.   1 2 3 4 5 6 7 8 9 10

16. My wife and I have a good marriage partnership.   1 2 3 4 5 6 7 8 9 10

17. I blame my wife for our problems.   1 2 3 4 5 6 7 8 9 10

18. Our closeness will not change when the kids leave home.   1 2 3 4 5 6 7 8 9 10

19. My marriage doesn't seem to have much purpose now.   1 2 3 4 5 6 7 8 9 10

20. I don't see why the kids get so much attention.   1 2 3 4 5 6 7 8 9 10

SCORING

Now add up the sum total of your circled numbers and your squared numbers and enter them below:

◯ Circled Score: _____   ☐ Squared Score: _____

A comparison of your scores can be obtained in two steps:

1. Compare your own current and wished for scores on each statement.
2. If a difference of more than twenty points exists between your *total* current and wished for scores, refer to the corresponding Metacare Guidelines in Chapter 12.

Chapter 8

DISENGAGING FROM HER

Having examined his "old identity" and purposes for continuing marriage, the middle-aged man often finds little reason to preserve his marriage. The principle of disengagement takes an early and perhaps commanding position. They move apart. James Kavanaugh gives us some insight in his poem "To Begin to Live the Rest of My Life" [1]

It makes no sense to my friends back home
That a middle-aged man should want to roam.
But I left the money and a share of fame
And I called it quits in the business game;
I left a house and a proper wife,
To begin to live the rest of my life.

It makes no sense to my swinging friends
That a middle-aged man should begin again.
So the stories grew and the rumors rolled
As the tale of my madness was oft retold.
But I can bear the gossip's knife
To begin to live the rest of my life.

It makes no sense to society
That a middle-aged man would take his leave.
The briefcase boys just shook their head,

My mother said I was better off dead.
But I packed my bag without advice
To begin to live the rest of my life.

It makes no sense to my neighborhood
That a middle-aged man is gone for good.
The preacher bowed his head and prayed,
My father said I should have stayed,
But I went away with the rumors rife
To begin to live the rest of my life.

Well I'm lonely now but my heart is free,
I enjoy a beer and watch a tree,
I can see a cloud and feel the breeze,
I can buy some bread and a bit of cheese.
And I know full well it is my right
To begin to live the rest of my life.

Now I have no plans for security,
No proper wife can depend on me,
I'm not too sure of eternity
But I know when a heart is really free.
And I walk along with a step that's light
To begin to live the rest of my life.

Like James Kavanaugh born in the minds of many middle-aged men are specific metathoughts such as "We are different people," "I can't be a divorced president," "I want romance," "Use it or lose it." Let's examine each of these metathoughts and then look inside several forms of disengagement such as an affair, separation, and divorce.

"We Are Different People"

While basic personality characteristics are probably less changeable after twenty or so, why would we assume we are married to the same partners at forty-five as we were at twenty, and if the partners change, doesn't the relationship?

A man consumed by his teak desk and nameplate at thirty

may suddenly become interested in sailing when he is fifty. The 1966 Mother of the Year might be known as the top credit manager for the local bank a dozen years later. Unable to recognize our changes, we go around blissfully assuming each partner is a Victorian fixture. Occasionally we will ask, "How come you didn't set the clock?" or "Why do you want to sleep on my side of the bed?" But change isn't built into our thoughts of marriage. "For ever and ever" appears as an immutable relationship.

A partner can change in yet another way. One partner may change while the other reinforces the past. She can reinforce the Barbie doll of yesteryear or the Mother McCree image; he can buy his retirement watch at forty-five and watch his career clock run out. She can wear her Levi's to the theater, while he comes to the dinner table in his motorcycle helmet.

"The Kids No Longer Need Me"

Separation and divorce reach a peak the year one's last child enters college. Often the metapausal man feels his child-rearing responsibilities are over then. He sees an empty marriage as well.

Other middle-aged men react differently. They wonder how much their marital warfare affects their children at home, whether it's worth for-better-or-worse. One day, they decide the answer is no. It's better for the children if they split. Some research confirms that children who live in homes full of conflict suffer more than children whose parents divorce. Lee G. Burchinal studied the personality adjustment characteristics of seventh-and eleventh-graders who came from intact homes, divorced homes, and remarriage homes. He could find little difference among them.[2]

"Amalgamated's Nonpresident No Longer Needs a Wife"

This reason for opting for sudden divorce makes sense to the middle-aged workaholic who, throughout his twenties, thirties, and early forties, has over-identified with his work. To be a successful executive, he needed a good cook, a wife who looked great at banquets and who made friends with fellow workers' wives at the country club ("Sally is a great help to me"). One day he realizes he isn't going to be president of the company. Guess what happens to Sally?

As his interest in work wanes in middle age, and dreams of being president hold less allure, so does the marriage he perpetuated as a tax write-off. An affair, separation, or divorce is the next step for him.

"It's Just No Good Anymore—I Want a Romance"

Many men have rather high romantic expectations from marriage that plummet dramatically in mid-life. Peter Pineo says that about 60 percent of his sample of middle-aged men were most disenchanted with demonstrations of affection and intimate relations in their marriage. He states:

Among these late divorces (mid-life), it is the magnitude and speed of their disenchantment which most fully characterizes the husbands.[3]

"Use it or Lose it!"

Waiting for the stop sign at Oak Street, the middle-aged man stares at the bumper sticker on the car ahead of him: "Use it or lose it." He reasons anew that his marriage isn't enough. He thinks back to the last time. . . . One middle-aged man said he had to write down what he did last month so his entire repertoire of techniques won't slip away between the sheets.

Preoccupied with a need to reaffirm his identity sexually, he waits late at night or until payday, hoping "tonight's the night." His inordinate need to check out his sexuality, coupled with the increasing rarity of his sexual activities, heightens his Gray Itch.

Today, the middle-aged man finds it impossible to get "intimate time" together, time to be close. He drives one hour a day, works ten, sleeps eight—1 + 10 + 8 = 19. He averages one hour a day on stop-sign committees, meetings, PTA; one hour a day playing with the kids; one and a half hours a day with TV; 1 hour a day eating. What's left: one-seventieth of his day for her!—or, at best, about 10 minutes a day or so.

Affair, Separation, or Divorce

For some, further disengagement occurs—an affair, separation, or a divorce is the result. We will examine each of these in the next sections to get a better look at the Gray Itch.

The Affair

The affair is a common means of disengagement from marriage by the metapausal man. Notice how in the story below a particular sequence of events develops in Earl's thinking about his wife. Notice also how he begins to redefine who he is in a new, exciting, and intimate relationship.

This new and excited image of who he is takes the pressure off the relationship at home—for he has someone else. He has a new yardstick of himself, someone who constantly tells him how nice he is to talk to or how good he is below the belt. To be close again has an overriding magnetism, a magnetism that draws him away from home, disengaging him further. It must be remembered that for men like Earl, a basic and overriding assessment of marital satisfaction is directly tied to demonstration of affection and intimate relations. Listen to his story:

One day, at a bar, someone else steps into my life. Ann could listen to me for hours, doesn't mind my belly, has a nice body, and really cares for me. She enjoys many of my favorite activities and, unlike my wife, Gerry, has nothing to do with the business enterprise at home.

Well, what is Ann really like? I don't know what she's like, and that's part of the enjoyment. She's attractive, but not beautiful. She, too, seemed lonely. As we talked, I noticed how she paid attention to me. I sat a little higher in my chair. She actually looked at me while I talked. I felt important. My discussion became more animated, more free. To make a point, I used my hands with as much assurance as the director of the Boston Pops. I suddenly recognized how starved I had been for communication. I jabbered on and on, rattling away like a runaway train. Even my old high school quips and more contemporary Polish jokes left her in stitches. She interrupted only one of my dissertations on the rotary engine to explain how much she liked talking to me. I haven't felt so important since the time I explained my indoor plant varieties to a Southern Illinois women's club.

Then, we left each other, but her parting comment was, "I could talk to you for hours." As I drove to Oak Street, I had a thought, "I didn't do anything wrong."

I struggled to say something at dinner during the family show-and-tell, but then I began to make the first in a long line of comparisons. Ann returned to my mind about 1:00 A.M. She remained with me until 5:18 appeared on my digital clock, my last recollection.

A couple of weeks went by. I had thoughts of her constantly like those that appear as light frames from a strobe light. I had to call her for lunch. The day before our lunch, I went shopping and bought a new shirt with extra-long collar points so I could wear it open at the neck. I took my new shirt, folded it carefully and placed it in my golf bag, waiting for the big day.

At the restaurant, I waited anxiously—I was embarrassed. Running through my mind this time weren't cute jokes or subjects such as rotary engines, but more serious matters.

Ann arrived and after having some difficulty finding my name on the reservation list, joined me. "Your name isn't really Namath, is it?" she asked. We sat side-by-side in a dark part of the restaurant. That day I held my knees together so I didn't touch hers.

There we sat. She commented on my shirt, which didn't look too wrinkled under my coat (too bad my golf bag isn't bigger). A bottle of wine loosened up my knees, and we talked and listened. Only Ann wasn't into talking about rotary engines that day. She talked about what she liked. "I really like spinach, too," I responded. I was surprised to hear her say that she loves skiing. She bent over toward me to show me the last signs of her goggle-marks from Vail. As she talked, two more metathoughts came over me: "I feel good" and "We have a lot in common."

Then, it's back to Oak Street. A week later, I called her for our third encounter. We forgot about our knees, I even grabbed her hand. As I did, my hand slipped into the relish dish. We both laughed. She doesn't care if I got pickle juice on her hand. I compared her to the other woman in my life, the one who doesn't like pickle juice.

That day the menu was more than liebfraumilch. It was a discussion of loneliness. "How can two people be married all these years and not understand each other?" Ann asked. "What is life for, anyway, other than to be close to someone?" she continued. And I said, "Yeah." "Pete [her husband] isn't bad, but he thinks I'm a hausfrau and seems to always be working. He's a workaholic," she said. And I said, "Yeah."

Our conversation moved from how she likes bald men to how lonely her friend is—poor Sally. I knew she wasn't really talking about Sally, so I countered with an anonymous "friend" of mine named George. Ann loved fixing artichokes, which happen to be George's favorite vegetable. Conversation on similar activities and foods, a need to care, and a hollowness inside, rolled into a hell of an afternoon. Before I knew it, it was 4:00 and I had missed the staff meeting again.

Now what? I asked myself on the way to Oak Street. Her hand was so warm, and her dress—nice body. Leaving off my shirt at the laundry under the name of Namath, I suddenly said, "Why not?" I called her for lunch again, put a deposit on Room 148 at a local motel under the name of Namath, and hoped.

By mid-afternoon, I was looking at Ann's body, sharing what I felt we both needed—intimacy. The trip to Oak Street that evening was sad for me—a mixture of leaving and coming home. Countless visual images of Ann, mixed with my feelings of guilt, continued as I caught myself watching my wife reading across the room that evening.

I continued to meet Ann occasionally for lunch and talk; to enjoy each other's bodies. Ann began to act as a sounding board for my pent-up feelings and questions about myself. She also confided in me.

A rationale began to build for Ann and against Gerry. My rationale went on and on. I caught myself saying, "If only Gerry had paid more attention to me. All she thinks about is her women's club and the kids. Ann needs me to talk to. I can help her.

My counterpoint comparisons, constant over the months, closely honed this rationalization. Each time I returned to Oak Street, I ran through the rationale as justification for my actions—Gerry is a bitch sometimes (not recognizing that I hadn't said a warm or decent word to her for several weeks).

Over the months, the guilt lessened and I became better in bed. Better? I was like a kid in a candy store. Middle-aged fears were nowhere in sight. Then those afternoons began to lap over into my staff meetings. Short images, over and over again—a body, a place—appeared in the budget sessions—and suddenly I was called back to reality by the president, who said, "Earl, Earl, can't you hear me? Your baselines are wrong—pay attention, will you?"

More guilt, a few lies, to stay at home or not to stay at home—and, then, back to Room 148. I fudged my expense account, pretended to be building new clients, and continued my affair. The rationale also continued to build. Gerry had given me a lot of good years. But Ann gave me something that Gerry no longer gave. "Maybe that's where it's at," I said to myself. "No, forget Ann—go home. How about the kids?"

I stopped at a local bar one day to think about Ann and missed another important meeting I had on the calendar. The constant transitions from the warm bed in Room 148 to 250 Oak Street were taking their toll on me, preoccupying and confounding me beyond reasonableness.

One night, unbelievably, I found myself walking around the house, twirling the key from Room 148 that I had forgotten to turn in. Fortunately, no one saw me. Then, I knew I had to do something. By now, I had acted so badly toward my wife that she was beginning to suspect. The family budget was continually poured into new sport shirts and more Grecian Formula."

I told Ann it was over, but we would keep in contact. I really felt guilty, and now I was alone. I lost that one person who was telling me I'm okay.

Then, one day, Ann told me she was separating from her husband. She also told me she was in love with me. I loved her, too, in a way, but I didn't know if I could commit myself to a lifetime with a 30-year-old. I tried to stay home, but like Thomas Wolfe said in *Look Homeward Angel,* "You can't go home again." It was over at home.

We see in Earl's story many standard characteristics of affairs of metapausal men. It's possible there is as much of a lockstep ritual to having an affair today as there is in the engagement process. Let's summarize part of the ritual.

1. The metapausal man in need of excitement finds someone to help redefine who he is.

2. An exciting person enters his life at this particularly vulnerable time.

3. Lunch and conversation lead to interesting communication about: (a) general things, (b) similar activities and vegetables, and (c) then loneliness, and (d) the need for intimacy. The latter is couched in third-person terms: "I have a friend who. . . ."

4. He feels important; someone is actually listening to him. Walking out of the restaurant, he feels good having his arm around another woman; it's exciting!

5. Comparisons begin between two women; between the afternoons in Room 148 and the evenings at 250 Oak Street.

6. He feels good about himself, even in a wrinkled shirt.

7. In Room 148 during an afternoon without a telephone, hair rollers, or kids coming in on him yelling, "My guppy died, Dad," he has an exceptional experience.

8. He feels like a pro in bed. It's exciting.

9. Then, a rationale develops, directed at his previous love object. This insidious script exaggerates his wife's faults in his mind. He says; (a) "Gerry doesn't understand me, (b) "I feel great with Ann," (c) "Ann needs me," and (d) "Gerry forced me into it."

10. Preoccupation with Ann affects his work; he begins boozing more.

11. He breaks it off with Ann, only to go back, based on a larger and more convincing rationale against his wife. He and Ann try it away from each other for a while as an important part of building that rationale.

12. He thinks it will last forever, but someone makes a move: (a) Ann leaves her husband, which puts him in a "put-up-

or-shut-up" position, or (b) his wife (or Ann's husband) discovers the affair.

13. He goes home, possibly rekindling love with his wife. For those who return, there is sometimes an improvement in the marital relationship following an affair, with one or both now more aware of their needs or desires to reconstruct the marital relationship.[4] After an affair some have increased sexual satisfaction within marriage. Now they are emotionally closer; the affair strengthened the marriage by turning the partners back toward each other.

14. The conflict that exists between two women he loves, his responsibility and freedom, and the obstacles before him appear as a challenge to his very manhood. Denis de Rougemont has stated:

Romance feeds on obstacles, short excitations and partings. Marriage, on the contrary, is made up of want, daily propinquity, growing accustomed to one another. Romance calls for far-away love. Where then, a couple has married in obedience to a romance, it is natural that the first time a conflict or a temperament or a taste becomes manifest, the parties ask each other, "Why did I marry?" and it is no less natural that, obsessed by universal propaganda in favor of romance, each should seize the first occasion to fall in love with someone else.

15. He separates or divorces.

Separation

Separation is a more frequent alternative for the middle-aged man with the Gray Itch who wishes to disengage from his marriage. It is also a logical next step after an affair. But since the American family has a thing about being together, the suggestion of separation has several difficulties.

André Gide, the French novelist, said, "Families, I hate you." He was rebelling not against the function of the family

but against its claim upon his total individuality, whole love
and interest. French historian Philippe Ariès says

The American nuclear family demands physical commitment to itself,
utilizing emotional bonding as its assumed glue. This bonding
together is a relatively new family concept.[7]

So, two things are true, First, many middle-aged men know
they don't feel emotionally bonded. As a matter of fact, they
are starving for some emotional expression. Secondly, they
have little training in expressing their emotions. They often fail
at the last vestige of the earlier marriage purpose, that of
providing emotional intimacy, and separation occurs.

Here's what Cliff told his counselor about what happened
after his separation:

Cliff called a few old friends. All agreed that they should get together,
but they always had to find a way to arrange schedules first. They
always seemed too busy. His boss and even his grown children also
withdrew from him as sanctions against his act. One day at the end of
a short telephone call from his daughter he asked her in deperation if
she wanted his telephone number. She said, "Just put it on your
Christmas card, Dad." That would have been all right, but it was July.
His daughter had no idea who he was, or who was at fault in causing
the separation. The fact that he moved out on his marriage was
enough.

In addition to a renewed emotional life full of women, Jack
Daniel's, and every conceivable kind of sports activity, Cliff also
hopes to get to know himself a little better. He really has little
knowledge of who he is or where he is going. Those points of earlier
identification—his wife, community, friends, a place, children—all
have suddenly disappeared.

Several possibilities for renewed identity occur to him. He can
become a workaholic, for he still has his trade. But this is a time when
he isn't into his work as much as he used to be. Still optimistic, but
somewhat battered by the newness and late hours of his activities, he
reassures himself by trying to have intercourse with every female in

sight. But most of it isn't very satisfying. Sex is easy, but people don't want to be close.

He's a hit in the office, however. Coworkers nudge him during a meeting and say, "Hey, how is it?" He smiles and usually says nothing. The envy of the office just plays it cool.

He's even tried the bar scene in the Marina. He is alternately therapist, spectator, and hunter. The therapist who sits in the bar always analyzing everybody and judging who has penis envy or who's schizophrenic. The spectator or voyeur who sits aside or toward the back and fantasizes but never does anything. Or the hunter who's constantly stalking his prey and, under the guise of intimacy, gathers marks on the wall to satisfy his insatiable hunting instinct.

And then Cliff goes through a period of being Grand Inquisitor—his own. He is constantly doing a number on himself. "Why do I feel this way?" "What should I do?" "If I do this, what about that?"

Eventually, evenings alone occur more often. As do contemplation and a preoccupation with "What should I do and where should I go?" From here, someone new steps into his life or he attempts to go home.

Divorce

This represents the last form of disengagement for the metapausal man. The incidence of divorce is greater in mid-life (ages forty to forty-four) than any other time, except during the first two adjustment years.[8]

As the ultimate "excuse" or weapon or concession or reason, divorce becomes a traumatic and complicated act for the middle-aged man.

Like the engagement and affairs process, the divorce process as a form of disengagement has a predictable set of steps.

Take the case of John:

John was a reasonably well-married man, at least that's what his wife Sally thought. Graying, to be sure. Less sure of himself—but married. One Sunday morning he suggested they skip church. He brought her coffee to bed along with the Sunday paper. Inserted within it were other papers—those for divorce.

Stages of Divorce

Paul Bohannan has postulated a set of divorce stages that

offers some insight into this form of the middle-aged man's
disengagement.[9]

Stage 1: Emotional Divorce. Throughout this book we have
seen each marriage partner assume that because he or she
shares a tube of toothpaste, the emotional glue that keeps a
marriage together will always be there. This sense of false
security lulls partners into not recognizing changing needs.

Arguments become weapons to attack each other's self-esteem.
A bill unpaid becomes a cheap shot; the way the other looks or
acts, a federal case. How to vote ends in a destructive episode
about the other's stupidity. In the twenty minutes a day
allocated to "us," destruction reigns. During the death march of
a marriage, the frail and hungry ego often surrenders, and
feelings become those of bereavement. The final burial cere-
monial, divorce, appears the only way out. As Barbara Strei-
sand sings, "It's over, all over." While divorce lies ahead, the
real last rites, emotional death, took place months or years ago.

Stage 2: Legal Divorce. Larry was a 51-year-old self-
employed businessman who was getting a divorce:

He entered the courtroom with his attorney whispering and coaching
him. As he walked down the aisle, he wondered if it was really him.
Twenty years before, he'd walked down the aisle and felt a great deal
different from today. The coaching from his attorney came into his
mind: "Don't say any more than you're asked. For heaven's sake,
don't tell them about your affair. Tell them your income varies from
year to year and this last year it was exceptionally high."

At the end of the aisle, as was true 20 years before, sat a woman
whose arms he'd had around him a few months before. Now she was
surrounded by attorneys, briefs, and bailiffs. Now instead of lovers
they were adversaries.

As the heavyset bailiff asked everyone to stand, Larry rose, only to
think how ridiculous it all was, arguing over kids you both love,
paying attorneys half a year's salary because you can't talk to each
other about money. The whole question of visitation rights was up for
grabs, as if one had to buy a ticket to see the only person in the world
who looked just like him.

Her attorney got up and claimed mental cruelty. And his attorney got up and said, "No contest." They divided up the pie—the lawn mower to him, the station wagon for her. He kept his retirement fund, and she kept the china. And it was over.

He had been judged free, a mythical condition that meant they both were alone, poor, and confused.

Stage 3: Economic Divorce. Economic divorce is probably a misnomer in the minds of many a middle-aged man. His reactions often range from saying, "Let her have it all—I'm moving to Florida," to saying, "I'm really gonna make that bitch pay." Beyond giving up what is partially his, the real problem is in setting up a second household, child support, alimony, and dividing up the investment pie.

First, taking old towels, his bar tools, and his clock radio, he moves out. By the time he stocks his new pad, he's broke and unable to put gas into his new sports car or take the next-door neighbor to dinner. After the attorneys get finished, he gets half of a color TV, his old golf cart, and a rare old picture of his grandmother. Left with the legacy of payments to the orthodontist for his daughter and tuition for his eldest son, he becomes bitter.

"Why did I work so hard all these years?" he says. "This must be worse than the crash in 1929." But he isn't finished yet. His wife, who complained for years about wanting to work, suddenly can't work a lick and becomes quite content with her one year of college. Legally divorced but economically encumbered, he feels like a teenager without wheels.

Stage 4: Bohanan writes further about Co-Parental Divorce. Waiting or calculating over the years when would be the best time to leave home in terms of the kids, the middle-aged man has great difficulty making the decision. There isn't a good time, although some times might be better than others. Regardless of who is at fault, he feels guilty because he is gone from the home, physically gone. His own striving to be free of a bad marriage is strangely coupled with his possessiveness. After all, his kids are his kids. Unable to recognize that people raise kids and not grow them, he exaggerates his loss into, "The kids can't survive without me."

Comments in the middle of an argument between teenage son and divorced father, such as "Don't tell me what to do—you don't live here anymore," momentarily rekindle his shame, guilt, mourning, and loss. Finally, as his guilt recedes, he begins to realize that it's in the best interest of the kids and they are not possessions, moved and directed by an absentee landlord. His thoughts of who has the final word in the matter of child rearing begin to have a logical answer. Instead of final authority, he becomes a consultant in such matters. This passive role stretches his personal feelings of manhood. His anger peaks the first time his ex-wife says that her boyfriend, Sam, feels he shouldn't punish the older son. After a while, anger melts away and what is best for the kids survives. Co-parental divorce becomes more of a reality.

Stage 5: Community Divorce. Trying to understand the middle-aged man in this stage of divorce, family and friends react in odd ways. In-laws say, "Well, he moved out, didn't he?" or "I knew he wasn't good enough for Alice from the start. Think about the poor children." From his own side of the family he gets more support, but deep down in the hearts of his aging parents is anxiety. They wonder what will happen to their grandchildren after the divorce.

Over the years, grandchildren have become a surrogate reason for living for his parents, offering meaning to them, a way for them to remain teachers. The divorce is also a divorce for them. Many a middle-aged man thinks, "At least I should get some support from my own parents," only to be shocked by their feelings of loss about their grandchildren.

Friends are also part of the community divorce. The Oak Street gang recently had its annual bash, but he wasn't invited. Friends don't like to get in the middle of it, and ignore the middle-aged man when he needs them most. Having cast off kids, wife, and house, he needs empathy, at least for a while. Unfortunately, friends, many of whom are also on the brink or insecure themselves about their own relationships, offer little help. He runs into the Oak Streeters eating dinner at a local restaurant before proceeding to another party. "I've been meaning to come and see you at the Marina," one calls from across the restaurant, and he says, "Sure, anytime," knowing full well that if the first one does, he'll get cut off for at least a month.

Gradually, the sense of loss of community pulls into perspective, for new friends are developed and possibly a new community. But initially, the quiet of one's apartment at night seems an inadequate substitute for the noisy dinner table he once found uncomfortable.

Stage 6: Psychic Divorce. This is closely related to the first stage, emotional divorce, with some unique qualities. Loss of a love object often leads to sleepless nights alone in a king-size bed in that $400-a-month apartment with the mirrored walls. This loss exists until a significant other is allowed to revive the wounded ego. Then, visits to Oak Street become more pleasant, indicating greater psychic divorce. He finds his ex isn't as castrating as he thought. Guilt, loss, mourning, and anger are left at Oak Street as he drives away. And it is amazing how he can function at work without wanting to take a punch at the competition or the boss.

Questions about whether it was all his wife's fault become "maybe it was both our faults." Introspection continues beyond a period of self-doubt, and a new sense of autonomy is spawned. Thoughts of the ex-wife in bed with another, how she can pay the mortgage, and how the kids are going to get along, fall into perspective, and divorce finally becomes complete.

As partners disengage, an affair, separation, and eventually divorce become a cause of pain within the metapausal man. He has an affair, separates, returns to his family, or breaks away permanently in his search as described previously by James Kavanaugh's poetic line, "And I walk along with a step that's light, to begin to live the rest of my life." The gray itch leads the middle-age man in search of a new or expanded "me"; he struggles with these events in hopes freedom will bring a new identity. Metathoughts of "Should I stay or leave home" often torment him until a decision is made.

H.I.M.M.
(Hallberg Index of Male Metapause)

AN AFFAIR, SEPARATION, AND/OR DIVORCE

The following statements should represent some of your present and future feelings and concerns about an affair, separation, and/or divorce.

DIRECTIONS

Please mark each statement twice. First, mark with a circle one number for each statement to represent your nearest current feeling about the subject. Second, mark one number with a square to represent where you would wish to see yourself regarding the statement. Higher numbers should equal stronger feelings.

EXAMPLE

I want to be somebody
other than the roles I play.   1 2 ③ 4 5 6 7 8 ⑨ 10

ABOUT AN AFFAIR, SEPARATION, AND DIVORCE

1. I am really a girl-watcher.   1 2 3 4 5 6 7 8 9 10

2. I don't have to love a woman to make love to her.   1 2 3 4 5 6 7 8 9 10

3. I often catch myself acting in ways I don't want to.   1 2 3 4 5 6 7 8 9 10

4. I don't care what others think about my divorce.   1 2 3 4 5 6 7 8 9 10

5. I like to do my own thing.   1 2 3 4 5 6 7 8 9 10

6. I like to take a risk.   1 2 3 4 5 6 7 8 9 10

7. I'd like to do something exciting.   1 2 3 4 5 6 7 8 9 10

8. I would feel guilty if I had sex with a woman other than my wife.   1 2 3 4 5 6 7 8 9 10

9. I would really like to have an affair if nobody found out.   1 2 3 4 5 6 7 8 9 10

10. I would like to separate from my wife but I can't afford it.   1 2 3 4 5 6 7 8 9 10

11. If I divorce, I'll never remarry.   1 2 3 4 5 6 7 8 9 10

12. I wish I could find someone to love me.   1 2 3 4 5 6 7 8 9 10

13. Romance is for kids.   1 2 3 4 5 6 7 8 9 10

14. I wish I had a little adventure in my life.   1 2 3 4 5 6 7 8 9 10

15. If I divorced, I would really miss my kids.   1 2 3 4 5 6 7 8 9 10

16. What would my family say if I asked for a divorce?   1 2 3 4 5 6 7 8 9 10

17. It must be exciting   1   2   3   4   5   6   7   8   9   10
to live in a singles
apartment house.

18. A lot of my divorced   1   2   3   4   5   6   7   8   9   10
friends are happy.

19. My wife and I are   1   2   3   4   5   6   7   8   9   10
fighting all the time.

20. My sex life is really   1   2   3   4   5   6   7   8   9   10
spontaneous   in
terms of time, place,
and manner.

SCORING

Now add up the sum total of your circled numbers and your squared numbers and enter them below.

◯ Circled Score: _____ ☐ Squared Score: _____

A comparison of your scores can be obtained in two steps:

1. Compare your own current and wished for scores on each statement.
2. If a difference of more than twenty points exists between your *total* current and wished for scores, refer to the corresponding Metacare Guidelines in Chapter 12.

Chapter 9

WHO CALLS THE SHOTS

Confused as some middle-aged men may be, they have never questioned their manhood in relation to the changing role of women until now. Today rigid, traditional roles designed by Zorba, Spartacus, and Joe Namath are full of chinks, heavy to carry, hot to wear, and probably out of date.

To see how role changes are actually affecting men, let's look at two types of vignettes. Each is related to the changing definition of womanhood and manhood and the changing identity of metapausal man. The first set of vignettes (1–3) are from recent counseling sessions, and relate to a definition of machismo; the second (4–6) relate to a rapidly changing set of female roles that affect the middle-aged man.

1. We'll listen to Jim, who has less get-up-and-go at work. Jim is a grocery store manager who is now fifty-two years old. He was known as a go-getter, a man of action. Jim was rarely found spending much time talking.

"I'm a doer," he said to a friend, "and I'm as strong as I always was." He could still lift several cases of string beans with one hand. He could stack faster than anybody in the chain. And figures? Nobody around could calculate price and margin as rapidly as he could.

But lately he has found himself forgetful about the margin and even the prices. "I'm doing all right. I don't need to watch all the prices as closely these day." He has trouble getting up for work. "I can't seem to get with it these days. I daydream more often—even while I'm checking out customers' groceries. I'm as strong as I ever was. But being on the go-go-go doesn't have what it used to for me. I'm wearing down," he explained to a friend.

2. Stan's decisiveness and positiveness are slipping. In a heated discussion, Stan's seventeen-year-old son said, "Dad, you don't know what you're talking about." Angered by his son, Stan just stood clenching his fists. Two years before, he would have knocked his son's block off, but now Stan was not sure what to do. He finally just walked away. Later, Stan really got mad at himself. "No kid of mine is going to tell me off," he thought. But Stan seems more passive and less aggressive these days. "I'm losing my ability to be boss around here" is a thought that bothers him. "In fact, I'm not looked up to at work as much these days. I ask too many people their opinions before making a judgment. I suppose I appear kind of weak to the younger fellows in the office."

3. We find Larry concerned that his logic is giving way to emotion. "Now Helen, I know how you feel about Lucy," Larry stated, "but logically it doesn't seem right that she would do that to you. If you think about it, it just doesn't make sense." This is the way Larry talked several months ago to his wife. But today he didn't. "It didn't even sound like me when I said, 'Helen, you must go with your feelings about Lucy.' Why did I get so involved with the way she felt?" Larry asked himself. "I guess I'm reading too many of these touchie-feelie books. I used to be the logical, scientific one in the family."

These three vignettes are indications of traditional definitions of manhood which are under question and changing. Jim was conditioned from a very early age to be active, strong, quick. He now finds these aspects of manliness are less important. Stan's father once had absolute control over his family. Now Stan finds himself walking away from his son's challenge, which later angers him tremendously and adds to his sense of identity confusion. We find Larry talking about feelings to his wife, something he recalls doing rarely.

These personal questions in metapause are related to another point of view. Middle-aged men use females in their lives to define what masculinity *is not*. How can he use as a reference point the female policeofficer who pulls him over or a female jockey who wins the daily double? Each throws his "I'm-not-her" outlook into a tailspin.

It's important that we look at some of the confusion that develops in his "I'm not her."

4. Tom's Sir Walter Raleigh role shattered as he hurried to hold the office door for a fellow office worker. As Tom graciously held the door open with one arm extended, the department secretary merely looked at him with indignation and walked through the door without a word. Tom wondered if it had been his breath. "Not a word. She didn't say a word," he muttered to himself.

5. Tim's provider role is threatened by his wife's career. Sarah bursts into the front door of the home she has shared with her husband for 17 years and says, "I got it! I got it!" "You got what?" he asks. "That job in Cleveland, silly," she responds. "But we live in California," he gasps.

6. Harry, a fiftyish computer executive, loses his image of the fairer sex to a sexually aggressive woman. Harry was in Los Angeles for a conference. Being new to the area, he asked a fellow conferee where the action was. He was led directly to a place called The Saloon in Beverly Hills, where he met a beautiful blonde. She looked like Candice Bergen and Ann-Margret put together. After a few drinks and some idle chatter, he tried to get up the nerve to ask her to dinner. About the time he was ready to ask, she leaned over and coquettishly said, "Do you screw?" As his face registered a sly, cool, "You bet," his testicles disappeared into the pit of his stomach just as they had the time he fell on the handlebars of his bicycle years earlier.

These last vignettes are only a few examples of countless shifts in the female role today that affect the middle-aged man's "I'm-not-her" maleness.

Historical Manhood and Traditional Womanhood

Probably the easiest way to understand maleness in America is to look at the stereotypes of both maleness and femaleness.

The middle-aged man was raised and conditioned in the 1930s, 1940s and 1950s to become masculine. Not only did the middle-aged man model his maleness after his father, uncle, friends, and favorite big-league pitcher, he also held traditional womanhood as a model of what *not* to be. A father modeling as a warrior nearly forty generations ago was not enough to make a man of his son. This modeling was assisted by his wife, his opposite, to create the necessary mirroring for his son to become a hero in the Roman legions; thus, we find a set of continua depicting maleness and femaleness as important sex stereotyping. These can be seen in the following list of male and female trips.

TABLE OF MALE/FEMALE TRIPS

Male Trips	*Female Trips*
Logical	Emotional
Dominant	Submissive
Competitive	Cooperative
Physical	Helpless
Sexual	Coquettish
Moneybags	Spiritual
Practical	Impractical
Strong and Silent	Sharing and Open
Independent	Dependent

A review of these stereotypes may assist the middle-aged man in determining the pressures and confusion related to his male image. Let's look at traditional malehood—machismo—and historical womanhood—fast becoming as extinct as the dinosaur.

The Logical Male versus the Emotional Female Trip

How many times have you caught yourself saying, "Let's not get emotional about it"? This statement is the result of a traditionally assumed female proclivity that has been conditioned out of most men from a very early age. Weren't you the one who made fun of the girl in the fourth grade who could multiply faster than the boys in your gang? Don't you do the bills? Don't you sign first in communications with the IRS? Most of us have been raised knowing how many miles it is between certain places. We remember how much the washing machine cost four years ago, don't we?

The opposite of you, the level-headed, logical man, is the stereotypical emotional woman. "How do you feel?" is a woman's question, isn't it? Women aren't very logical, are they? Only women cry, right? Like Gable and Leigh in *Gone with the Wind*, the male and female are mirror images in this logical/emotional continuum.

The Dominant Male versus Submissive Female Trip

Remember on the playground how the girls used to wait for you to organize the game? In high school *you* decided where to go with a date. And aren't final decisions in the family made by you? "Let your father decide" was heard in most families as the middle-aged man grew up. Even though you may logically resist authoritiarian behavior, you feel justified in shouting orders.

On the other hand, her stereotype represents a submissive trip. "Whatever you say, dear," she's told you for years, or, "Ask your father, he'll know what's best." Whenever the great warrior wanted his dinner or his bed, he got it from her, for surrender and compliance were marks of her womanhood.

The Competitive Male versus the Cooperative Female Trip

Historically, manhood has been encrusted with the dubious honor of being competitive and being the aggressor. From the time you drew a line on the playground that few others crossed, to feeling frustrated and helpless on your back while a beautiful woman makes love to you, you, the middle-aged man have been conditioned to be aggressive. At the office you demon-strate your aggressiveness through a clipped, decisive voice and a field general's strategy to ruin the opposition.

On Saturday you put on the old number 64 sweatshirt, striped crew socks, and tennis shoes and attack the front lawn with the zest of a Dallas Cowboy. Except for a World War II movie, the Friday night fights, and karate exhibits, you really hate television. Marc Fasteau points out in a recent article:

The male machine is a special kind of being ... different from women, children and those men who don't measure up. He is functional, designed mainly for work. He is programmed to tackle jobs, override obstacles, attack problems, overcome difficulties, and always seize the offensive. He will take on any task that can be presented to him in a competitive framework. His most positive reinforcement is victory.[1]

His opposite is the female stereotype—the cooperative trip. The woman acts as the family mediator and assists her man. She prepares dinner for the eastern regional sales managers, is careful not to let her interests compete with his. Because she's emotional, submissive, and cooperative, she would be lousy at meeting the competition.

The Physical Male Trip versus Helpless Female Trip

Even at a time of life when your body begins to look like the object of kick-the-can, you still press the body trip. You run two miles each morning and collapse in your lover's arms in the evening, saying, "I'm too tired, dear." You wear jeans so tight you get nauseous when you bend over to look at the bathroom scale. You're the kind of guy who in the fourth grade tripped little girls or tried to see who could spit the highest up over the principal's door. You feel ego strength is a new form of international weight lifting.

Thinking about her, you wouldn't consider arm wrestling with her. When you start a tennis match, you always give her a two-point advantage, don't you? Doesn't she bring the pickle jar to you to open? Isn't she supposed to be physically helpless—and you her knight in shining armor?

The Sexual Male versus Coquettish Female Trip

The traditional male tests his manhood every time he gets into bed. Success in bed equals winning; he's still a man.

On the opposite end of this continuum, that nice girl you married wasn't very experienced, was she? Her definition of femininity and yours involved a female who was supposed to be good in bed intuitively, but without practice. The reason for these strange expectations were that you were—in the old days— allowed to have sexual experience without love, but she wasn't.

The Moneybags Male versus Spiritual Female Trip

Many middle-aged man translate their machismo into dollars and cents. In some parts of the city, they drive around with a TV antenna on their cars. In other parts of the city, they drive with a CB radio aerial. At work, they drive for a larger desk, the largest office on the highest floor, and more money as definitions of success.

At home, you transmit your moneybags trip to the kids by giving each of them ten dollars after having an argument with them. To the oldest son who needs to talk to you, you give the Bank Americard for the evening out. As old Daddy Warbucks, your checkbook in mid-life has taken on the value of your jock size in an earlier time.

While the male thermometer of success is often the number of bucks he makes each year, the female is not supposed to be interested in money. Higher values, spiritual things, caring for and raising children, going to church—these are the ways of a woman. She drives the older car, rarely goes out to lunch. It isn't that the traditional woman didn't like to spend money; she did. It just wasn't equated with her womanhood.

The Practical Male versus Impractical Female Trip

"I'm the practical one in the family," you tell a friend. "Yeah, last month my wife even wanted to join a church, but I told her that it was too far to drive. 'You've got to be more practical, Sally,' I told her. 'You know, I don't buy anything that can't help me.' The other day, Sally came home with a Matisse print and I said, 'What good's that going to do us?' "

The American male is supposed to be the practical one in the family. The impractical partner is, obviously, his opposite. How many times in the past have you told her, "That isn't practical, honey," and she just backs up into her old stereotype, smiles, and says, "But women aren't supposed to be practical, dear."

The Strong, Silent Male versus the Sharing, Open Female Trip

Here we find the traditional middle-aged macho male tied to the quiet, silent type. He bangs his head on the door and says little. He cuts his hand on the kitchen knife, only to report, "it's nothing," as the blood fills the sink. "I'm all right," he says as he falls on his son's skateboard in the driveway. Yet, as he gets up, a voice inside says, "That really hurt."

He sees a gripping movie on TV. A small tear appears in his eye, but he wipes it off and tells his wife that it's only the smog. Throughout his life, he's been unable to cry for fear of being a "crybaby" or a "sissy."

A friend recently witnessed his two-year-old son falling on the deck of the cabin during a summer cocktail party. The father immediately said, "Get up! Get up! Don't cry! Don't cry!" A couple of hours later, his young daughter fell on the same spot. As she began crying, he picked her up and held her close to him throughout the rest of the party. The conditioning based on sex was obvious.

If you're a man, you don't tell others how you feel, do you? One of the most tangible problems in counseling middle-aged men is their inability to disclose their feelings. After several sessions with these men, it's interesting to see how many of them open up to each other. Some of them report, "I haven't felt I could really talk to another man since I was in high school."

In *The Hazards of Being Male,* Herb Goldberg discloses:

In the course of interviewing adult males, I became particularly aware of the isolation of many of the married ones. While most men denied being lonely, they almost all indicated that their wives were their only close friend, the only person they really trusted. They blamed their lack of friends on being too busy but the real reasons were significantly more complex than that.[2]

The Independent Male versus the Dependent Female Trip

Part of male machismo is also related to the area of independence. Males are taught to explore, stand on their own two feet, and be independent. This sense of strong independence has been the subject of many counseling sessions concerning affection and intimacy within a marriage. Some counselors have reported that this sense of male independence disallows deep affection and intimacy.

On the other hand, dependency was part of the definition of the traditional woman. The weaker sex, submissive, more emotional, less practical, she needed to depend on somebody. Women traditionally were supposed to follow their males around the way a right cornerback checks the tight end. She was supposed to have her bags packed and change-of-address cards already stamped when her husband came home and announced that he'd got a new job in Jersey. Dependence was part of her identity.

We have found, then, that the traditional male and female identity trips seem to develop out of a series of opposite stereotypes of what a man *is* and what he *isn't.*

Metapausal Male's Confusion

For the better part of forty centuries, middle-aged men have known these differences between girls and boys, men and women. Then, one day, somebody invented the washing machine; then came the Pill, and ten years later there was a revolution. What Women's Liberation is or has done has been well documented elsewhere, but what it means to the middle-aged has not been.

In the midst of this revolution, we find the metapausal man's manhood changing because of the shifts in the new female trip.

Except for a few Archie Bunker types, the American male feels, in his head, that some Women's Liberation's a good thing. However, in many ways, he has not been able to adjust emotionally to the transitions that are necessary for him to see this as reality. He's confused when he enters the room where final negotiations for a contract are to be held. Thinking, as he enters, that he can hold his own with those bastards from Consolidated, he finds that Consolidated's representative is a honey-haired, green-eyed beauty, ten years younger than he, with two more college degrees, who is also tough as nails. He loses the contract.

Imagine the middle-aged man sitting by the TV drinking a beer when his wife says, "George, I'm going back to school for my Ph.D." Imagine him seated on the hard bleachers on a spring Saturday witnessing his twelve-year-old daughter making a perfect hook-slide into second base, something he could never do. Imagine him as he telephones for the time and hears a low, masculine voice respond, "When you hear the tone, the time will be . . ." Even Monday night football is no exception—the female sportscaster tells him what's going on in the huddle. Our middle-aged man goes to New York on business, enters a small bar, and has a fleeting thought about cutting in on a couple dancing, but is unable to discern which of them is the female. His confusion in the bar exists all through the familiar refrain of Helen Reddy's song, "I am woman", in effect she's singing "I Can Do Anything Better Than You." His golf club has a lady's day, but wouldn't dare to have a men's day. And the corporation has a beautiful thirty-year-old vice-president with nice tits who is after his job.

Sometimes he wishes he were old instead of middle-aged. He wouldn't have to cope with these confusions.

He doesn't like frozen TV dinners or his wife selling real estate at night. He fumes when, instead of their sailing, her term paper must be done. He's bored at all this talk about equality and Women's Liberation. At a time when the middle-aged man needs a clearer navigational system, he can't tell which pair of Levi's in the closet are his.

The following counseling cases show us some of the meta-pausal man's resistance to the women's movement.

Sam explained in the following case about some of his territory, his logical versus her emotional side. His real agenda relates to his fears about how he and his wife are changing.

Sam: You know, every time I used to argue with her, she'd cry. I'd try to reason with her and she would tell me I was cold and calculating. Then, in frustration, I'd yell at her and she would start bawling even more, and leave the room.

Counselor: What's wrong with her crying?

Sam: Nothing, I guess—women do it. I knew where I stood then, I knew how far I could go in an argument, but now, now. . . .

Counselor: Tell us about what's happening now, Sam.

Sam: It's funny. We were arguing politics the other night in front of my folks. She stood in there tenaciously with an opinion. She was logical and probably right, but I didn't like her to do it.

Counselor: To do what, Sam?

Sam: Well, the next thing you know, she'll think she's as good as I am. (He laughs.)

Counselor: Stay with the subject, Sam.

Sam: Okay. I guess I felt she was stepping into my territory. You know, many men are still telling their wives how to vote and how to logically figure out who the candidates are and what they have to offer.

Counselor: They do?

Sam: Yes. And, look, I'm not as physically strong as I used to be, but I'll be damned if I'll give up. I'm really sharp about politics too, and she's got to recognize that.

It's easy to see Sam's trip about being the logical one is a partial substitute for his declining physical prowess.

An Atlanta computer salesman points out his own conflicts:

Len: I've never been very romantic myself. That was always my wife's department.
Counselor: Why was it her responsibility?
Len: Well, you know how women are, crying in the movies, sending flowers to friends.
Counselor: You sound like you feel that's the way it *was*. Is that correct?
Len: Yes. For the first time in my life, I feel like romance—probably because I want something more than what my work has given me. Last year I started growing bonsai, and I really enjoyed it. And I didn't feel like a sissy, either. But, more important, I need romance. Today a couple of guys at the office are having affairs, and I envy them. Long lunches, someone exciting to be with. But I feel guilty thinking about it and asked my wife to go away for the weekend with me, instead. You know, someplace up the Coast.
Counselor: What did she say when you asked her?
Len: She said, "Fine," but when she looked at her calendar, we couldn't find time to go until June. And it was only March! Can you imagine that? She reminded me also that I had promised to change the sprinkler system on the front lawn, and to paint under the eaves before the summer. That really irritated me.
Counselor: Why?
Len: Because, because I *need* romance now, and all I got from her were realities of life. We really switched roles. You know what she said to me? She said, "Len, I'd love to go, but how much do you think it will cost?" Crap! I'm in the mood for romance, and she's into the budget. I just got up and walked out of the room saying, "We'll put it on the BankAmericard." And her answer followed me all the way into the den: "Len, the BankAmericard is over $1,000 right now."

Fred, a separated auto mechanic in the Midwest, tells his group how he feels about the shifts in his macho trips and his girl friend, as they affect his sex life:

Fred: The other night, she even told me, "A little higher"—can you believe it? As if I didn't know.

Counselor: Yes, Fred, but if she had some place she wanted you to be—

Fred: I know, but it's as though all of a sudden she got on top. I felt like I was the student and she was the teacher.

Counselor: Fred, so you feel you should always control the performance in the sexual activity?

Fred: Well, not really, but it's different. . . . I like her to be aggressive and do different things sometimes, but I think I should initiate them.

Counselor: That doesn't exactly make sense, Fred. Can you elaborate on that?

Fred: Say, it boils down to the fact that the man is supposed to direct the act.

Counselor: Why, Fred?

Fred: Because he's more experienced, knows more about it.

Counselor: Was your girl friend a virgin when you first met her, Fred?

Fred: Yes.

Counselor: She's not a virgin now, Fred, is she?

Fred: I know . . . but . . . if she gets *me* excited, I lose control. I have to see to it she has an orgasm, don't I? I can only do that if I have control.

Menopause

Beyond the general revolution occurring within our partners today, the middle-aged man must contend with yet another change—menopause.

Some women report that during this experience they notice no change, and some that they feel a wrenching psychological as well as physiological change. To better understand his own changes, the middle-aged man must recognize what occurs in his partner during menopause.

Tim had difficulty understanding menopause. "Sarah's impossible to live with," Tim said. "Just at the time I have the chance to become vice-president, she can't attend any of the company parties. She gets nervous, says that her skin is all creepy. And guess what? She has to sit by an open window most of the time. Imagine! In December—how ridiculous. She's just trying to give me a bad time. She even says she can't sleep at night and keeps me awake. What a time for my wife to flip out."

Two basic and important areas of menopause must be misunderstood by Tim and other middle-aged men. The first one is the cessation of menstruation itself, which is commonly called menopause, and the other is the psychological and social changes that are more aptly called the female climacteric.

Literally, the word *menopause* means "the end, pause of the menses," or monthly bleeding. When used precisely, this term refers only to the permanent ending of menstruation, which occurs because the ovaries become depleted of eggs and hormone-producing cells. In normal women of reproductive age, the ovaries produce a hormone, estrogen, in certain amounts throughout the monthly cycle. In middle age, a gradual decline in the periodic release of estrogen occurs, mainly between the ages of forty-eight and fifty-two.[3] However, menopause may occur abruptly, causing certain psychological traumas as well as physical change.

The female climacteric is the second area. It includes psychological, social, and psychosomatic changes in the middle-aged woman much like metapause changes in the middle-aged man. The term *climacteric* comes from a Greek word meaning rung in a ladder, to indicate a step or a change in the person's life. The climacteric is more commonly referred to as the woman's "change of life." A significant increase in the changes associated with the climacteric occurs between the ages of forty-five and fifty-four.

Myths about Menopause

We might further improve our understanding of what happens to our partners in menopause by looking at another area that molds the middle-aged man's thinking about her (and about himself)—the myths about menopause:

1. *Women aren't interested in sex after menopause.* While it can be documented that after thirty-five a gradual decline in sexual interest does occur in both males and females, there's little or no evidence to indicate that a sudden or dramatic drop in sexual interest occurs. There is no evidence whatsoever that the normal, healthy woman is no longer interested in sexual intercourse during or after menopause.

2. *"My wife is always depressed during her period."* "When she skipped a period, I really had to tread lightly." Several points need to be understood here. First, there is a small amount of evidence indicating that males as well as females experience a cyclical mood cycle during a monthly or six-week period.[4] Much of these mood swings may be attributed to the changes in the amount of estrogen and other female hormones secreted during woman's monthly cycle.

   However, menopause doesn't seem to be a major reason for the "treading lightly," much as she doesn't need to tread lightly with you.

3. *"My Alice is really testy these days as she goes through menopause."* Again, with the secretion of male hormones during menopause in women and a decrease of estrogen and other female hormones, some females will take on more of the male characteristics as they age. The converse is also true of men. Through clinical observations, Jung has suggested that, as people age, males become more female-like.

   Many women become more tolerant of their own aggressive and egocentric impulses and men more tolerant of their nurturant and affiliative impulses.

4. *"Since our kids went away to college, Eve has been less interested in our marriage."* This myth actually contradicts what we know about marriage satisfaction levels after the launching period of children—that is, when children leave the home, many marriages improve.

   Most of the evidence in this area indicates that there is a general improvement in the satisfaction of each partner after this launching period. It is true that directly after children leave home there is a condition called "the empty-nest syndrome." This syndrome appears to both fathers and mothers as a void in their lives. The quiet within the household, the fact that the family car is actually parked in the driveway and the budget is in the black for the first time are all concomitants of this empty-nest syndrome.

The middle-aged man's identity is deeply tied to his own feeling of machismo. His manliness has been learned through the development of a set of male-conditioned trips as well as their opposites, the female trips. The metapausal man is confronted with the major revolution of this decade and possibly of this century—the shifting role and liberation of women. And he must deal with another shift that takes place in women during mid-life, menopause. All this occurs within one of the important mirrors of "Who am I?"

H.I.M.M.
(Hallberg Index of Male Metapause)

WHO CALLS THE SHOTS

The statements that follow should represent some of your present and future feelings and concerns about your relationship with your wife or lover, as it relates to metapause.

DIRECTIONS

Please mark each statement twice. First, mark with a circle one number for each statement to represent your nearest current feeling about the subject. Second, mark one number with a square to represent where you would wish to see yourself in the future regarding the statement. Higher numbers should equal stronger feelings.

EXAMPLE

My wife and I aren't
close anymore.   1   2   ③   4   5   6̲   7   8   9   10

SHOTS STATEMENTS

1. I want to be some-body other than the roles I play, such as husband or com-pany man.   1 2 3 4 5 6 7 8 9 10

2. I don't like things to change too fast.   1 2 3 4 5 6 7 8 9 10

3. I feel uncertain about myself these days.   1 2 3 4 5 6 7 8 9 10

4. I wish to return to the good old days.   1 2 3 4 5 6 7 8 9 10

5. It would bother me if my wife made more money than I do.   1 2 3 4 5 6 7 8 9 10

6. I like my wife to be partially dependent on me.   1 2 3 4 5 6 7 8 9 10

7. I really feel I'm the scientific one in the family.   1 2 3 4 5 6 7 8 9 10

8. I would not be con-sidered very ro-mantic.   1 2 3 4 5 6 7 8 9 10

9. I have encouraged my wife to go back to school.   1 2 3 4 5 6 7 8 9 10

10. My wife is really menopausal lately.

1 2 3 4 5 6 7 8 9 10

11. I seem to be the emotional one in the family.

1 2 3 4 5 6 7 8 9 10

12. I think most men will gain from Women's Liberation eventually.

1 2 3 4 5 6 7 8 9 10

13. The trouble with Women's Liberation is it makes women too independent.

1 2 3 4 5 6 7 8 9 10

14. What happened to that soft, warm girl I married?

1 2 3 4 5 6 7 8 9 10

15. My wife has really changed in the last three years.

1 2 3 4 5 6 7 8 9 10

16. I feel more affectionate these days.

1 2 3 4 5 6 7 8 9 10

17. I believe in women having a career.

1 2 3 4 5 6 7 8 9 10

18. My wife feels my career is more important.

1 2 3 4 5 6 7 8 9 10

19. I don't like these new women who are aggressive.

1 2 3 4 5 6 7 8 9 10

20. It's more difficult to-   1 2 3 4 5 6 7 8 9 10
    day to maintain
    your manhood.

SCORING

Now add up the sum total of your circled numbers and your squared numbers and enter them below:

○ Circled Score: _____   ☐ Squared Score: _____

A comparison of your scores can be obtained in two steps:

1. Compare your own current and wished for scores on each statement.
2. If a difference of more than twenty points exists between your *total* current and wished for scores, refer to the corresponding Metacare Guidelines in Chapter 12.

Chapter 10

HAS ANYONE SEEN MY FATHER?

That young person who looks something like the metapausal man and talks like him through the surfer haircut or smiling braces *is* him—or so the middle-aged father thought. Reflected in this seventeen-year-old is the middle-aged man's ability as a provider, teacher, and lover. When he says, "That's my girl," or, "He's just a chip off the old block," Dad is not merely talking of his children, but of himself. For years, when things got rough at work or with his wife, his reasons for continuing were justified in one saying: "Think of the kids." Not only did the kids add to dad's original purpose, but they also influenced his behavior—his Levi's suit, his use of "foxy" and "super."

As the young are important to the middle-aged man's identity, so are those family members older than he, his parents. To a lesser extent, he is still influenced by "What would the folks say?" as much as "What would the kids think?" Watching his parents age reflects upon his life cycle as well, and his impressions of death.

As parents and kids change, the metapausal man develops a cloudy misunderstanding of each generation. Suddenly, meta-thoughts crowd in from one side of the generation gap. "The kids don't need me anymore." "Sue will finish law school next year." "Bruce is going to move away from us after he gets married." "Everything I say just seems to go right through him." And on the other side, another gap: "I must visit my mother this week." "My folks are getting older." "My father seems a little more forgetful." Examining these double-edged generation-gap mirrors may give us some additional insight as to causes for the male metapause.

A Chip Off the Old Block

Tim is a forty-nine-year-old assembly-line foreman who tells his counseling group about his estrangement from his children. Tim was driving up Oak Street at the end of the day, as he had for the last ten years. The day had been too much. As he entered the front door, he found no one there. Years before, the whole family would have converged as he approached, chattering as they came. Bill would have looked up at him and pulled his legs; Mark would have elbowed him to play football on the front lawn, and the baby would have crawled as fast as she could toward him. All would have been talking at once, asking about his day. He would have responded after giving them each a hug and a kiss. Tonight as he moved through the house, he hurdled seventeen-year-old, fourteen-year-old, and ten-year old bodies sprawled in front of the TV. As he passed, two bodies grunted an imperceptible greeting, while the third didn't even look up from the TV. He could have been the Boston Strangler, and she wouldn't even have noticed. Lying on the floor, holding her head in her hands, she reports, "Mom said you would barbecue chicken," and, "Dad, remember this is the night for Mom's class. And Dad, don't forget to do the bills tonight." He sidestepped three half-eaten bowls of ice cream sundaes, five shoes, two sweaters, and an algebra book on his way to the refrigerator, where he thrust in his hand to dig out a beer.

Indignant, he thought to himself, "These kids would probably pay more attention to the meter reader. "What am I doing? What am I, a father or a baby-sitter?"

During dinner, each of the four around the table tried to talk to each other, but it was like being at a UN debate. Mark talked of how rotten our government was and of his calculus problems. On one subject, Tim disagreed, of the other one, he knew nothing. Bill talked of his tennis practice. Tim was envious; his game was atrocious; he never had time. And the baby, although now ten, talked of how her friends were "getting it on." Then she talked about the chauvinist pig who teaches her history class and uses *his* instead of *his and/or her*. At a precise point, the dinner ended, sounded by a belch from Mark. All split from the table. The roars of Mark's Chevy van, Bill's stereo in his room, and Jill's TV indicated all were in their places. The family evening was over.

Later in the evening, with his beer next to him, he tackled the bills. He couldn't believe that the miscellaneous account added up to the national debt.

During his bill-paying, he metathought: "The kids seem so indifferent toward me; they take me for granted." "Why can't I talk to the kids anymore?" "They make me feel envious and yet mad." "Buy, buy, buy—they have no conception of money." An additional metathought streaked through his mind: "Why do I feel like a foreign exchange student in my own house?"

So ended another day at 711 Oak Street.

In Tim's case, his self-identity becomes shaky when reflected in the differences of values and beliefs between him and his children. Every time he says "black" the kids say "white." One says "the establishment this-or-that" and he says, "When I was your age. . . ." He's losing his hair, and his daughter's is so long that it sticks out below the bottom of her parka. He's flabby, and his son puts his fist through the side of the garage. He works; they watch TV. He wants to talk to them, and they barricade themselves in their rooms or take off in their vans. He likes *Time* magazine; they read *Rolling Stone*. He likes quiet music, and they like rock propelled by 100-watt stereo systems. He saves for college; they don't know if they want to go. He likes a drink at night, and they talk about how many of his brain cells will be destroyed. His oldest smokes pot, and Tim quit smoking 10 years ago.

He can't utilize his "prides and joys" as navigational points to know where he is in mid-life. While he's sometimes fearful of these changes in his relationship with his kids, he epitomizes the cool, staunch member of the community, an emotional rock. His feelings and his fears rarely show.

Maybe we can help the middle-aged man understand how his identity is slipping if we look at adolescence, and differences in beliefs and communication between generations. In *Culture and Commitment,* Margaret Mead points out that a father cannot evoke his own youth to understand the young:

At this breaking point between two radically different and closely related groups, both are inevitably very lonely as we face each other, knowing that they will never experience what we have experienced, and that we can never experience what they have experienced. Once the fact of a deep, new, unprecedented, world-wide generation gap is firmly established in the minds of both the young and the old, communication can be established again.[1]

Adolescence

Adolescence is an interesting and conflicting time, a time to just sit around and listen to yourself squeak and grow. In fact, the concept of adolescence is fairly new. Up until 100 years ago, there wasn't even a definite period called adolescence. Most young people worked on the farm or in the factory beginning at age 8 or 10. The distance between a father and his adolescent son was lessened by the fact that they worked shoulder-to-shoulder in the field or in the shop. Each was dependent on the other. The son learned the trade from his father, and the father required the work of his son to advance his holdings or his craft. There was a natural perpetuation of the craft from father to son, and each mirrored the purpose in which the other was intrinsically involved.

Under patriarchal rule, differences between generations existed but because of mutual dependence rarely broke into open warfare. When warfare did occur, the son was often banished.

Today the conflict is different. Due to our technology, parents play a smaller part in educating youth. Tim was actually unable to understand his son's calculus. Due to this same technology, special trades call for special degrees, and the young are forced to continue their training or preparation for nearly one-third of their lives. Thus, adolescence is often entended for an exaggerated length of time. The rewards of adulthood are held on increasingly longer carrot sticks—high school, college, graduate school. Today males are able to get the rewards of the society—marriage, political affiliations, money, and status—only after their sexual drive has begun to decline. It seems quite strange and twisted that one is only able to buy into a declining market.

We have seen part of our problem. On the younger side, adolescence creates an "I'm-not-you" reaction toward the father. On the other side, reactions such as "When I was your age" represent a continuous desire to mold the young into what the middle-aged are, not only because the metapausal man feels it is best, but also because it is all that he knows.

It should be obvious to the middle-aged man that his kids are *not* growing up to be like the old man any more than he wanted to be just like the boss who took him under his wing or like his own father.

Competition from his son such as when his son beats him at tennis or arm-wrestling comes precisely at a time when both are unsure of themselves, the son in adolescence and the middle-aged man in metapause. Both are seeking a new identity, the younger man trying to carve out a "me" and utilizing his father as mirror, and the middle-aged man keying off the younger in his search for a new "me" in mid-life. Each is jockeying for position in a sea of rapidly changing societal values and conflicts, causing communication difficulties.

Different Beliefs

Belief differences between generations occur in the minds of the young because they seek different interpretations of their values than their fathers'. Let's examine some of these important differences:

Experience

There are several differences between the way kids and parents look at experience. The metapausal man values experience highly and tells youth that experienced people are wiser. And yet youth questions whether wisdom always follows experience. Trust is placed in their own first-hand knowledge and not that of Dad.

Individuality

Individuality is the second area of belief where major differences occur. On the one hand, the middle-aged man tells youth to "be yourself"; yet, the grown-up worries about what other people think about his age, his appearance, his furniture, his clothes, and his home. What youth hears is that individuality is important; what they see is that his father has little confidence in his own uniqueness.

Freedom

In the area of freedom, youth insists, unlike his father, that freedom is a right and not a privilege, that you don't have to earn freedom by cleaning your room—it is a guarantee.

Responsibility

Responsibility is the next area. Here we find men at metacenter unwilling to give responsibility to youth so they can actually learn to be responsible persons. The youth wonders how responsibility can be learned without having the authority to make some of their own decisions.

These first four belief differences often cause misunderstanding between the middle-aged man and his son or daughter.

Work

The fifth area is probably the most important. As a company man, our hero slaves a twelve-hour day. For years his work has taken him away from his family on the 7:18, and he has returned late at night. The youth often feels that his father has lost his inviduality, his freedom to pursue pleasures beyond his work.

Youth often feels truth in the lyrics of Tim Buckley's "Goodbye and Hello" that describe antique people, godless and sexless, in our industrial civilization. They work in dark dungeons and worship technology and money while sacrificing their sons.

Materialism

Another area of belief which causes differences between middle-aged man's and his children's views is materialism. Everybody knows that money talks. But the extensive preoccupation with money and what money often symbolizes in our society causes great difficulty to the teenager in the family.

Education

Education represents another important area of disagreement. Many of us in middle age believe that a college education is the answer to most of our personal, occupational, and social problems. However, after twenty or thirty years of increasing college attendance by their predecessors, youth today are beginning to see that education itself is not the answer to all their problems. Major differences exist between the reasoning of the middle-aged man who puts money away so his son or daughter can go to college, and the seeming indifference of some youth about whether they attend college or not.

Morality

The last important area of belief differences is that of moral values. Subtle shifts in morality have occurred in some youth. They feel moral decisions are the prerogative of the individual, not of external authorites.

The Times They Are A-Changin'

Coupled with belief differences, social change affects the middle-aged man's identity with the younger generation. In four specific ways, social change affects our ability to relate to one another across the generation gap. First, change has made the world substantially different in time and place for each generation. New inventions, new philosophies, new problems exist that did not exist when the middle-aged man was young. Even if the middle-aged man and his kids live under the same roof, they live in different times and places.

Rapid change is unprecedented today. The British author, scientist, and lecturer C. P. Snow once observed, "Until this century, social change was so slow, it passed unnoticed in a person's lifetime." [2] In this century, changes have occurred rapidly.

Change can also lead to psychological frustration. Although youth encourages change, its results are not always psychologically positive. In the rapid pace of modern living, one can easily lose his reference points or his identifications. The outcome can be uncertain and result in loneliness and alienation for the young as well as for the middle-aged.

The fourth reason change affects us is the distance between technological change and its social fallout. Rapid technological change poses a special set of problems for the different generations. Think of the impact of the automobile, the bomb, space exploration, and the pill on our society. Think of the fact that possibly by 1989, five-billion people will live on this earth, populated in 1970 by three billion. Think about the fact that 20 percent of Americans move every five years. As Alvin Toffler has said, "Of the 885,000 listings in the Washington, D.C. telephone book in 1969, over half were different from the year before (and this wasn't even an election year)." [3] Can we see some additional disorientation of the metapausal man's navigational system?

Communication Difficulties

Due to changes in beliefs and rapid technological change, communication between the middle-aged man and his kids is often stressed. The actual amount of "getting through," or communication, may be very little. Paul Simon wrote about the "sounds of silence," and Fred Neal wrote a song called "Everybody's Talkin' at Me, and I Don't Hear a Word They're Sayin'." Each depicts the problem.

Dr. William Thomas and I studied the kinds of communication difficulties that occur between parents and their teenage children. We found that a number of key phrases and words cause tune-outs, which in turn disconnect the communication between parents and youth. Some of the most popular ones on the parent's side: "Take my word for it," "If you work hard, you will," "Someday you'll understand," "The trouble with your generation is . . . ," "When I was your age . . ." This last is the title of the Hallberg-Thomas book on the subject.[4] On the other side of the generation gap, youth says: "You're just part of the establishment," "You wouldn't understand," "It's not relevant," "It's different now, Ma." Each of these causes tune-outs.

Metapausal Male Stereotypes

Popular stereotypes of middle-aged men who have difficulty communicating with their children do exist. One is the *jellyfish:* This is the father who in mid-life is unable to say yes or no to anything. He brings to mind the old schoolyard game "stop-and-go." He's afraid to commit himself because he's unable to adjust to a changing world.

The second one is the *dictator.* We've all known dictators—they're the ones who are always lecturing or scolding. They're always right; they end the conversation with "right is right" or "we'll talk about it no further." The dictator has an opinion about everything.

Still another one is the *martyr.* "Oh, how we sacrificed! We gave her everything!" The martyr complex is a typical stereotype of some middle-aged men. The martyr would have taken a better job in another city if it weren't for the kids. "We'd have better clothes if we didn't spend everything on you," he says. "Look at how you made us suffer," he implies in a number of ways. Through guilt, the martyr tries to cling tenaciously to his son or daughter.

Then, of course, there's *moneybags*. Moneybags is always substituting money and presents for good communication, affection, and understanding. Moneybags tends to treat the young person as a commodity. After a family argument, he hopes to make up the distance between him and his son or daughter by offering ten dollars or the car keys.

The *one-armed paper hanger* is always too busy to talk to his kids. "Talk to me later." "Wait till I'm finished with dinner." "Don't bother me while I'm watching TV." "You see that I brought work home; let's talk about it later." This sort of tune-out infects the middle-aged man's vocabulary. Unwilling to deal with the problem or to listen, he attempts to offer his business or his involvement elsewhere as an excuse.

Then, of course, there's the *blamer*. This parent, whenever something frustrating or confusing comes up between himself and his son or daughter, has to look for somebody to fault. "It's the teacher's fault" or "It's your fault." "It's your mother's fault," he says. This pattern actually represents a fear of the responsibility for being wrong; it manifests a continuing need to relieve himself of the burden of involvement in something unpleasant.

The Older Generation

As the middle-aged man is taken aback by his problems with his children, he turns around to find yet another chasm, another gap—that of his changing perceptions of his own parents. At a time when the middle-aged man needs to search for a new and revitalized self, a new identification, possibly even a new freedom, the image of who he is in relation to his parents also fogs up. The middle-aged man not only has generated confusion with those he has sired, but also with those who have sired him. Of course this discomfort is not limited to men. Here's what one woman reports:

It is as if there are two mirrors before me: Each held at a partial angle. I see part of myself in my mother, who is growing old, and part of her in me. In the other mirror, I see part of myself in my daughter. I've had some dramatic insights just from looking into these mirrors. It is a set of revelations that I suppose can only come when you are in the middle of three generations." [5]

Still responsible for the younger generation and assuming more responsibility for the older, the metapausal man finds himself negotiating both sides of the generation gap. The older generation says, "They didn't do it that way in my time," and the younger says, "My time is now." The middle-aged man finds himself truly in the middle.

The metapausal man's father says, "This is the way it is," while the middle-aged man offers each of his children a vote as to how he should spend his two-week vacation. As a child, the metapausal man was seen and not heard, whereas in his own family, everyone drops everything to listen to the children.

Kenneth Soddy tells what it means to be caught between generations:

The situation may be complex in the individual member of the middle generation, who may have some nostalgia for the old self-image as a member of the younger generation—maybe confronted by his own parents in the older generation and, what is more imponderable but may be a highly distorted influence by way of the memory of his parents at an age of which he, himself, now is. There are many possible sources of tension here.[6]

Added Tensions

For the first time in history, three vital, mature, and healthy generations exist at the same time. Each has its own power, autonomy, and opinions. Each, through its strength, causes communications difficulties and increasing identity problems for the middle-aged man.

The middle-aged man grows his hair longer, and his son tells him he looks like a California surfer. He buys a sports car, and his son feels he's just trying to "make it," and his father thinks he should have bought something more economical.

Most middle-aged men are obviously unaware of these differences and experience ambivalence as well as guilt about their aging parents. Conversely, the parents feel confused over their own changes in role and loss of power in the family. These several confusions set up communications problems between the two generations, as they do with the younger generation.

Tensions over Parental Modeling

In early life, the now middle-aged man modeled himself after his father by taking giant strides on a mountain trail, sitting in his father's chair, wearing his father's hat, all in hopes that the model of his father would show up in his own mirror someday. Later, as an adolescent, he looked at his parents as negative models—what *not* to say, how *not* to dress, and sometimes what *not* to believe. His parents seemed to have little value as models at that time.

Tensions over Added Responsibilities and Guilt

Now we find him at metacenter with mixed feelings about his parents. He respects their wisdom—but years of preoccupation with his own nuclear family have left his parents as near-foreigners within the greater family structure. For this he feels guilty. As his parents age, he must spend more time with them, time that he may wish to spend enjoying what he wants to do. For this he feels guilty. He now has to watch over them. His mother needs to put a towel rack up and calls him in the middle of a dinner party. His parents drop in to see him when he's late for his bowling league. He neglects to see his father in a retirement home. He either has his parents living with him or feels guilty if they don't.

This is particularly important when one of his parents passes away, for then the middle-aged man must play the role of a surrogate spouse as well as a son. He often takes on all of this new responsibility with an increasing amount of guilt.

Tension over Loss of Family Position

His father no longer controls the economics and doesn't even sit at the head of the table anymore. He probably isn't even involved in the major decisions affecting the family. Except for Colonel Sanders, the average eighty-year-old has little position and power in the American family. This leads to many tensions in the family.

A demonstration of loss of power is exemplified by the parent who meddles. Because he has less power, he tends to try to take over whenever he can. He'll say, "It's none of my business, dear, but. . . ."

Loss of Affection

Little affection is transmitted to the older generation by their children today, causing additional tension. The older person receives very little affection, while he is still expected to provide it within the family. How often have we seen an elderly person with his head on the lap of one of his children? A now-famous bumper sticker we see on Oak Street states appropriately: "Old men need love, too."

The middle-aged man knows that he doesn't demonstrate affection toward his parents, which also makes him feel guilty.

Feeling of Rejection

Aging parents' fear of rejection also produces tension between generations. Feeling rejected is a fear for all ages, but expecially for the elderly person.

Delayed Gratification

More family tension in mid-life is generated by long-delayed self-gratification. The middle-aged man begins to feel he has given up much in raising his children, and his parents feel he doesn't appreciate what they have done for him.

Increased Dependency on the Part of Parents

The middle-aged son feels an increased responsibility toward parental financial well-being. This at a time when his own family is in the launching stage involving college and weddings, and when he himself may be contemplating separation or divorce. The financial role of the son toward his elderly parents becomes especially trying and guilt-provoking.

Aging and Death

Mourning the loss of his own youth, the middle-aged man sees his future mirrored in his aging parents. For example, his aging parents' loss of memory becomes a potential loss for him. A flashback of a recent conversation where his father continually brought up experiences he had heard many times before emphasizes the problem. As their health begins to fade and their power in the family decreases, he looks at himself and says, "It's my turn next."

The identity or mirroring relationship between the middle-aged man and his parents cannot be understood fully unless we look at the final event—death—and its components, grief and mourning. His parents are a constant reminder to the middle-aged man of his own mortality.

In discussion groups with metapausal men, there's an indication of a wide range of reactions to life's last event. Joe held, "I haven't thought much about it. I'm too busy at work." Larry felt, "I don't want to be twenty again. I just want to enjoy the next twenty." And Steve also commented, "I never thought much about it until Ben, my partner, died on the golf course at forty-seven. God, that was depressing. He just kicked the bucket."

Attempting to ferret out and understand these reactions, we find a special consideration of death common among middle-aged men. The certainty of eventual death plays an important part in where the middle-aged man finds himself.

Death—the Final Fact of Life

The inevitability of death, a tangible event in our lives, is a fact often really discovered in mid-life. Everybody understands death as a concept. But truly recognizing that life, whether good or bad, has limits and is not infinite, gives the middle-aged man a paradoxical navigational point. Until mid-life, the slogan "You only go around once" was just a beer commercial. Now, in mid-life, the gusto must contend with despair. The middle-aged man sees his next sportscar or sexual act as his last. A special "I've-been-cheated" feeling can easily occur in the middle-aged man when he realizes he has a limited time left. A sense of urgency returns to him, an urgency similar to the need to break from his parents when he left for college. Wives comment on how the middle-aged man seems to mope around for a while and then he has to do everything "today." One wife said:

The family is so tired of his "you only go around once" activities. We just don't feel the urgency that he does. He goes to a party and is the last one to leave, just in case it is his last party. He drinks one extra for the trip home, like there's no tomorrow. He's so compulsive. Today he got reservations for a trip to California which is a year off. Last year, he would have waited until a day before we left. And, spending money. I used to be the extravagant one. Now, his BankAmericard looks like half the national debt, all due to a you-only-go-around-once philosophy of enjoy and enjoy, before it's too late. At his current frenzy, it'll be over before he can get the beer can out of the ice chest.

Another perplexed wife commented on how a wily motor home salesman caught her husband off guard as they walked out of the showroom. Recognizing a sense of urgency in this metapausal husband, the motor home salesman whispered, "You'll be pushing up daisies before long, why don't you give it a try?" That episode cost his family $204 a month in payments.

On the depression and despair end of the gusto-versus-despair continuum, we find some middle-aged men reacting to the discovery that death is inevitable by keeping their black suits pressed and hanging in a special place in the closet. Within this group, any pain from overeating lasagne to a lower-back ache causes him to put his safe-deposit box key under his pillow. This forty-year-old makes a fetish out of his aches and pains. He tells the kids to be quiet during a Preparation H commercial on TV. His favorite TV characters are the guys with the boxing glove and the hammer on the Alka-Seltzer commercial, and his favorite commercial is the guy with the red sinus cavities. It's so bad that the once staunch Republican begins to argue for Medicare at forty. His sinuses, which have always acted up, suddenly become diphtheria. His old football injury not only flares up the Saturday when the lawn needs mowing, but also when he's in the missionary position. Commiserating with a special set of cronies at the local bar, he drinks to each one's health and really means it. A few years before, this same group was drinking to all the beautiful women in the world, and meaning it. This desperation group sits around and mutters metathoughts like, "one hour is just another hour gone," or, "The past is gone," or, "I wonder what it's like—they say you don't feel a thing." Within this group, depression and mental illness can also be the result of knowledge that there are only two absolutes in life, and taxes is the least important.

Each of these ends of the continuum, then, causes middle-aged man's continual buffeting about the existential questions of life and death.

Caught between youth and old age, the metapausal man sees other shifts in who he is. His own flesh and blood seems different, their beliefs and communication foreign to him. On the other side of the generation gap, his parents age. As his responsibilities mount at home, his own parents require more of him. Through his parents he begins to look at death for the first time—not out of fear so much as out of the need to use his time from metacenter to death more efficiently.

H.I.M.M.
(Hallberg Index of Metapause)

HAS ANYONE SEEN MY FATHER

The statements that follow should represent some of your present and future feelings and concerns about generational concerns as discussed in this chapter.

DIRECTIONS

Please mark each statement twice. First, mark with a circle one number for each statement to represent your nearest current feeling about the subject. Second, mark one number with a square to represent where you would wish to see yourself regarding the statement. Higher numbers should equal stronger feelings.

EXAMPLE

I think about the death of
my parents quite often.   1 2 ③ 4 5 6 7 ⑧ 9 10

HAS ANYONE SEEN MY FATHER?

1. Upon my death I   1 2 3 4 5 6 7 8 9 10
   want to leave something important to my family.

2. I think about the   1 2 3 4 5 6 7 8 9 10
   death of my parents quite often.

3. I rarely talk to my   1 2 3 4 5 6 7 8 9 10
   kids, except about their school or my business.

4. My children rarely   1 2 3 4 5 6 7 8 9 10
   ask about my day.

5. My children's ado-   1 2 3 4 5 6 7 8 9 10
   lescence really confuses me.

6. I share leisure-time activities with my children.

1 2 3 4 5 6 7 8 9 10

7. I sacrificed to put my children through college.

1 2 3 4 5 6 7 8 9 10

8. I feel guilty when I don't visit my mother often.

1 2 3 4 5 6 7 8 9 10

9. I really miss not having the kids around the house.

1 2 3 4 5 6 7 8 9 10

10. I look forward to going home each night and being with the kids.

1 2 3 4 5 6 7 8 9 10

11. My parents are so dependent upon me these days.

1 2 3 4 5 6 7 8 9 10

12. I'm not very affectionate with my parents.

1 2 3 4 5 6 7 8 9 10

13. My kids seem better educated than I do.

1 2 3 4 5 6 7 8 9 10

14. I spend a lot of time thinking about my parents.

1 2 3 4 5 6 7 8 9 10

15. The death of a   1 2 3 4 5 6 7 8 9 10
    friend or family
    member really gets
    to me.

16. My kids don't listen   1 2 3 4 5 6 7 8 9 10
    to me.

17. I like a quiet evening 1 2 3 4 5 6 7 8 9 10
    at home.

18. I generally make my   1 2 3 4 5 6 7 8 9 10
    plans all alone.

19. My kids and my par-   1 2 3 4 5 6 7 8 9 10
    ents think I'm suc-
    cessful.

20. I'm really respected   1 2 3 4 5 6 7 8 9 10
    as a good father
    more than a corpo-
    rate executive.

SCORING

Now add up the sum total of your circled numbers and your
squared numbers and enter them below:

○ Circled Score: _____   ☐ Squared Score: _____

A comparison of your scores can be obtained in two steps:

1. Compare your own current and wished for scores on each
   statement.
2. If a difference of more than twenty points exists between
   your *total* current and wished for scores, refer to the corresponding Metacare Guidelines in Chapter 12.

Part III

YOU ONLY
GO AROUND
ONCE

Chapter 11

MALE METAPAUSE ASSESSMENT: Hallberg Index of Male Metapause (H.I.M.M.)

We've covered a lot of territory, shared our suffering, maybe learned more about what we're like as metapausal men. Our search of The Gray Itch has taken us through an exhaustive examination of the characteristics of metapause. Now it is time to assess ourselves, our own characteristics of The Gray Itch.

Before we actually start our Metacare Action Planning, we must discover where we are out of focus—and how much. What causes the double vision and how much of it can be measured in mid-life?

Let's imagine you've just appointed a manager—a manager of your own company—you are that company. And your charge is to get the company from the red to the black, from The Gray Itch to emansumated man (more about this later). What do you need to do? Well, first you've got to bring in a few new people to help you.

You need a vice-president for observation or assessment. This expert will assist you to observe your own actions, to help you. This V.P. will measure your behavior, observe and keep records about what you are like today and also ascertain what you wish to be in the future.

You also need to hire a vice-president for planning—the director of Metacare Action Planning.

Now, turn your company over to the vice-presidents—allow yourself to be assessed and a plan to be suggested. It's your company.

Hallberg Index of Male Metapause (H.I.M.M.)

The H.I.M.M. is designed to spotlight areas where the middle-aged man is metapausal. The series of metathoughts have been abstracted at the end of each chapter in Part II and represent your score in the most significant areas related to metapause.

A short review will get us started. You were asked to mark each item *twice*—once to represent where you are currently and once to represent where you wish to be. Identifying your personal feelings, you marked each item by *circling* the number closest to how strongly you feel *currently* about the position stated. Then you marked a number by drawing a *square* around the number that represented where you would *like* to be.

Some items may have seemed incomplete or vague; however, you were asked to select a position (number) that was relatively, most acceptable to you. There were no right answers, and there was no time limit. The stronger you felt about one statement, the larger the number was, that you marked.

Now you are ready to see where you stand.

Scoring the H.I.M.M. has four steps. Before beginning, be sure that you have circled *and* placed squares on the numbered statements after each chapter in Part II.

Step 1: add the total number of points signified by the *circled* numbers of each chapter. Enter your subtotal on the H.I.M.M. scoresheet that follows, under "Current."

Step 2: Add the total number of points signified by the numbers squared for each chapter. List the total number of points under "Wished For."

Third step, subtract or find the difference between your total "Current" and "Wished For" scores, for each of the seven areas. For each of the areas place the score differences under the column "Difference."

Fourth step, add up all your subtotal points from all the areas for the Current and Wished For calculations.

H.I.M.M. SCORE SHEET

Metapausal Index Areas	(Circles) Current	(Squares) Wished	Difference
1) Vice-President Who?			
2) Physical Me			
3) Sexual I.D.			
4) For Better or For Worse			
5) Disengaging from Her			
6) Who Calls the Shots?			
7) Has Anyone Seen My Father?			

H.I.M.M. Interpretation

A comparison of your scores can be obtained in two steps:

1. Compare the differences between Current and Wished For scores in each of the seven areas. Are there any large differences?
2. Areas where more than a twenty-point spread exists between Current and Wished For should be noted and you should refer to the corresponding Metacare Planning guidelines in Chapter 12.

Now that your vice-president for assessment is finished, allow your vice-president for planning to take your H.I.M.M. assessment and apply it to Metacare Action Planning.

Chapter 12

METACARE ACTION PLANNING

We have covered two important aspects of understanding The Gray Itch. We observed what metapause was in Parts I and II of this book.

In the last chapter we used our vice-president for assessment and the H.I.M.M. to see what we are like currently and where we would wish to be in the future.

Now we need our vice-president of planning, control, and willpower to move us beyond male metapause toward emansumated manhood.

1. Select those chapters where at least a 20-point spread or difference exists in your Metapause Index score between what you presently feel and where you wish to be.
2. Then read over the corresponding Metacare Action Guideline for each chapter.
3. Design yourself a simple Metacare program for each area.
4. Set aside a little time each week for 3 months to practice your Metacare program and prepare you for the next 20 or 30 years.

I. Metacare Action Planning Guidelines—Vice-President Who?—Chapter 4

There are several Metacare Guidelines that can change your lot at work.

A. *Keep work in perspective.* Believe it or not, the American male is not made just for work. He can enjoy leisure and individual interests. One of the saddest aspects of the middle-aged man is his inability to separate himself from his work, to get perspective. Being a workaholic is one of the most common problems he faces.

B. *Plan a work separation.* If you're a workaholic, plan for a partial separation. Develop a new interest or cultivate one of your old ones. Set some time aside for it each week. At first you'll feel like you're cheating on your true love (work). As with all losses, plan to have a mourning period, a period of loss for your work, cut back just as you did when you quit smoking. Years of carrying your briefcase home full of items has become your mid-life teddy bear. And it has been a way you've avoided family responsibilities by hiding out in the den. Develop a section in your briefcase for information about your new interest or leave your briefcase in the office once in a while.

C. *When should you rewind your career clock?*
Examine your career clock; check your career ladder.

1. Write down where you started and what your goals or advancements have been in 20 years. What do the floor and ceiling rungs of your career ladder look like today in reference to these stated goals of years before?

2. Do a scenario about your work. Write a review of your total career as if you were 70 years of age. What's different about what you have written and where you are today?

3. Add three promotions to your career ladder. Where will you be? Will you be bringing home that much more money? How much more time from your life will those new jobs take?

D. *How to change your work.* We have found that many middle-aged men feel trapped in their work, and yet several things can be done to improve their own personal working conditions.

1. Move toward more control and autonomy in your work. Try to take on projects where you have more control, such as devising a new merchandising program or a new territory. Management development personnel call this "plan-to-control," a technique for developing autonomy and pride in one's work.
2. Attempt to work with younger persons and try to teach them some of what you know.
3. Get involved in training or the selection of new personnel. Try to work toward leaving a mark on the company. This is difficult, but involvement in new programs or management programs is a possibility for you.
4. Job enrichment—attempt to add new dimensions to your work. You'll find the time if these are interesting new tasks for you, and you will be more efficient.
5. Job enlargement—try to take on some of the functions of your boss. A good boss will be happy to delegate to you, and you will find your job more exciting.

E. *Tuning into a second career.* With early retirement the rule for many middle-aged men, the development of a second career can be exciting and satisfying. Possibly you want one in which you are the boss and have more control of your destiny at work, such as running a small business.

Many middle-aged men and women are returning to school to study in new areas. You'll be afraid of the grade competition at first. But the evidence indicates that returning middle-aged students seem to do as well or better than younger ones.

F. *How to set new career goals.* Write three goals for your "second-half" career; place them on a time line; make them realistic. Can you accomplish them? What else would you like to do with the rest of your life?

G. *Preparing for a sabbatical.* The mid-life sabbatical is becoming more and more popular. Why should there be a moritorium on work only during adolescence? What's wrong with a middle-age backpacker in Europe or ski instructor in Aspen? Some can't afford time away from their work, but more can today than ever before. Possibly if you and your wife work full-time for a couple of years, you both can take a sabbatical. I know, you're too important to get away for a year. Well, try three months; then, at the end of that time, call in to talk to someone in your office. I'm willing to bet that the secretary, when taking your call, will say, "Bill who? Please spell your name."

II. Metacare Action Planning Guidelines—Physical Me— Chapter 5

Here are some Metacare Planning Guidelines to change your physical self.

A. *Have a heart.* Unless there's a special medical reason to, don't be overly careful about your heart. It's a strong, viable organ that doesn't atrophy with age as many other muscles do. Try not to be "oversensitized" to your healthy heart; it'll make an old man out of you nearly as fast as a heart attack. We have "overadvertised" heart disease and probably made all of us hypersensitive to the slightest pain in the left arm.

Like any other muscle, the heart needs exercise regularly and in moderate amounts. We can't expect to add a column of numbers as rapidly today, nor can we expect our hearts to adjust from 100 beats a minute to 200 beats the single time we jog each month. Regular to moderate exercise is what is needed.

Change your diet. Give up most saturated fats;
the evidence is overwhelming in this area. Any fat
that hardens at room temperature should be elimi-
nated or cut way down.

Avoid stress as much as possible. While the last
line of evidence isn't in, it does appear that stress
causes a long line of chain reactions that affect the
heart. Stress apparently constricts the blood vessels,
which in turn radio the kidneys to spew out
additional hormones, which further constricts the
blood vessels.

B. *Cosmetic changes.* I suppose with the exception of
false eyelashes, men today have involved themselves with all forms of cosmetics to change their
lives. Cosmetic changes can do little, however, to
make us a new or different person.

So if you feel you want to dye your hair, do it. If
you want a toupee, buy it and wear it. If they make
you feel better about your life, cosmetic changes can
be important.

C. *How much alcohol?* Remember, the highest incidence of male alcoholism occurs in middle age.
Alcohol definitely should be a limited part of the
middle-aged man's Metacare program. It exaggerates our depressions, it makes us fat, it cuts into our
sex lives, and it destroys our brain cells. All told, it's
an unwise drug to use in great quantities. However,
it tastes good and makes us feel good. Therefore,
don't give it up. But watch it!

Also, try not to use alcohol as a way of punishing
yourself or others in your life. Many of us whip
ourselves with doubles and triples. In many ways,
overindulgence in alcohol is a masochistic trip of
the middle-aged man.

D. How to reduce stress. The first thing to do is to
figure out your stress times. Each year there are
predictable stress times: income tax, annual reports,
weddings, or anniversaries. Place them on your

calendar. Try not to select these times to break up with your wife, fight with your kids, or plan a move to Seattle. Stress time can also run in monthly cycles. From the beginning of the month, when we need to pay bills, to the end of the month, when we don't have anything to pay them with, stress tends to increase and decrease in rhythmic cycles. There are stress times each day: making the train, those first few minutes in the front door at night. The major point here is that you can usually predict the stress points in your life and, through this recognition, *budget out your stress.*

While evidence for this is not extensive, a great deal of stress may develop in the middle-aged man owing to a conflict between "being somebody" and just "being." Many daydream about this dilemma and feel stress. Whether to be vice-president of the company or build a mountain cabin, attack a new client or enjoy lunch with an old friend—these questions gnaw at us and cause stress.

E. *Training your diet.* Many diets are possible. Most of them lead to rather dramatic results initially but are difficult to follow over a long period of time.

Here's a two-part program to overcome fat.

1. Select any of the standard diets you like and get down to the weight that you wish. Be careful to set a goal you can reach.

2. Develop a weight-maintenance program by doing three things:

   a. Give up four foods you often eat—entirely! Start with the junk foods—potato chips, cereals, Twinkies. But consider giving up some nutritional foods, too. One friend gave up milk and found that he could reduce his weight four or five pounds the first year. The average person in the United States eats 120 pounds of sugar a year. Imagine the calories in that much sugar! Don't give up any of your favorite foods, however. If you give up four or five foods that are fattening, your total caloric intake for the year will be reduced significantly, allowing you to maintain a weight level with as little pain as possible. The bottom line will be a yearly decrease in caloric intake and a drop in weight.

b. Have a talk with your wife and have her cut down on your food portions by about 15 percent. It's not much, but over a year's time that's a lot of bread and potatoes. This 15 percent reduction may be enough for the middle-aged man to break even with his decreasing metabolic rate. Also, ask her to serve dinners from the stove so that dishes of your favorite foods on the table do not demand that you take a second helping.

c. Cut down on the booze. The amount of calories in booze is extraordinary. One shot of booze contains only 100 calories. But who has one shot? Or even one drink these days? Besides, by the time you add tonic, grenadine, olives, cherries, and cream floats, and side dishes of crackers and onion dip, the amount of calories is unbelievable! And wine isn't any better. For the same amount of "effect" you get from whiskey you may need two or three glasses of wine, or approximately 500 to 600 calories.

F. *Staying in shape takes effort.* If you wish to tone up those muscles and decrease that shortness of breath, you must commit some time. If you don't want to spend the time, continue to look like a twelve-year-old Greek olive or last month's yogurt in a Glad Bag.

The muscles that appear to flab first in the middle-aged man are those that are not used. Chest and stomach muscles aren't very challenged behind a mahogany desk or sitting on the 6:18

to Connecticut. Some physical activity is necessary. An exercise program should include the following elements:

1. Buy yourself a twenty- to forty-pound weight and work up to twenty repetitions on your arms, stomach, and chest. Take approximately ten minutes a day for this exercise.
2. Situps are also important for the middle-aged man; approximately twenty a day are sufficient, requiring about 5 minutes.
3. Get an activity that's fun. Part of keeping in shape is your attitude. If you get involved with an activity you like, you have something to look forward to. Even tennis elbow makes for a good discussion at a cocktail party. Try to pick an activity with some adventure in it. Some of the best ones are skiing, sailing, tennis, golf, backpacking, and motorcycling. Forget the handball or basketball. By age fifty it's too much for you.
4. Take up running. Develop a jogging program. This is probably the most efficient form of exercise for you, for it only takes about twenty minutes a run. Try to run for ten minutes each time, gradually building up to two miles. You will notice improved respiration and a slight loss of weight. Don't run to lose a lot of weight. It's nearly impossible to do. After you build up to two miles, you will see your weight has dropped by five to fifteen pounds.

   You will also notice that running is boring as hell, but so are other parts of your life. Besides, how bored can you get in twenty minutes?

   Don't plan to run every day. Plan to run a set number of miles a week, six or eight, after you've worked up to it. Try to run with a friend, if possible. Conversation and the mutual pain make it easier. Plan to run at the same time, either in the morning or in the evening. This will

keep you on schedule. Morning schedules are an
easier running program, and an exciting activity
on weekends. You'll find that you will keep in
pretty good shape and look much better.

III. **Metacare Action Planning Guidelines—Sexual I.D.—
Chapter 6**
   A. *Psychological problem.* One of the greatest un-
   knowns about middle-aged males is the effects of
   their personal psychology on their sex lives. Many
   middle-aged men who show sexual dysfunction
   really are psychologically "sexed out." Countless
   cases of impotence in middle age are cured suddenly with a single affair.
      First and foremost, the middle-aged man must
   want sex and, on occasion, even take it (with
   permission, of course). A middle-aged man must be
   psychologically motivated toward sex. This implies
   that each partner must certainly remain interesting
   to the other.
      Fears of sexual inadequacy and the numbers
   game are often causes when the middle-aged man
   says, "I'm too tired tonight—I really worked hard
   today." This is the male equivalent of "I've got a
   headache."
   B. *How to conquer the intellectual problem.* With all the
   emphasis on technique, variety, and *Deep Throat,*
   it's a wonder any of us can make love. We
   constantly compare ourselves to the *National En-
   quirer,* Japanese watercolors, or those small, obscure
   ads for condoms in the back of *Playgirl* magazine.
   Thus, we approach our sexual partner as ana-
   lytically as if we were preparing to give an annual
   report.
   C. *Understanding performance requirements.* Stop trying to perform like the director of a cheap summer
   stock theater in New Hampshire. Your responsibility is not to see that the lights work, the actors are in

the right positions, the lines are learned before curtain goes up. Sex is not a recital; it's the emotional expression of two people. You're not in bed with the editor of an exposé magazine; there are no reviews; just express yourself.

D. *Deciding about the main event.* Sex is part of a loving relationship, not its goal. This may sound old-fashioned, but the problem is, most middle-aged men feel love is expressed only by a sudden overwhelming urge. If they compare sex to playing in the Super Bowl, of course they're going to worry about their performance. Forget about what's happening high above the stadium in the Goodyear blimp. Just make love to her. Sex is a part of the loving process, integrated into a total loving relationship.

E. *Play with her.* If you follow the above guidelines, you will finally be able to play with your partner. Remember how it was when you were on your honeymoon? How you laughed in bed, made love, tickled each other, had your head scratched. Well, if you want that psychological desire for sex to return, forget about that new position you've learned. Forget about the lighting for the main event. Think about sex as a play experience as well as a part of love. Sometimes just talk to her. You do not have a climax every time you tickle her. If you do play, your afternoons in bed will take on an intimacy you never imagined possible. It will bring out the child in you, and in her as well. Play is one of man's most satisfying behaviors. Share this real joy of life. Where else could you have an innocent, spontaneous, sometimes childlike, sometimes close experience in our society? In the boardroom? In the grocery store?

F. *Understanding malus erectus.* Male machoism doesn't equal an erection. If it did, most of us would be men for only a few minutes a week (if we're lucky). You can perform sexually in a playful, caring atmosphere and manner without needing to have the biggest one in town. Try to enjoy one of your greatest expressions without a scorecard. Who cares how many birdies or pars you get? Sometimes even be submissive; allow her to make love to you. Often this is difficult for men who feel they have to be on top all the time to remain manly, but you'll find it a joyful and not an emasculating experience.

G. *How to develop your own techniques.* We don't all write, walk, draw, spit, drive, eat, or belch the same way; why should we look like everyone else while we're making love? Whether you're a C– or an A is only relevant when you're in school. Set your own standards and invent your own techniques, but be careful, for whenever standards are set or techniques applied, you might start measuring yourself again.

H. *Select a new place.* Take her away with you at least once every two months. That bed you generally sleep in, even with your new closet mirrors, may not always be the place for lovemaking. We learned at an early age there was a place for everything: our toys, our napkins, our cars. But there really isn't a place for sex. In the sand at the beach, under a pine tree, or in a motel are just as appropriate and possibly even more exciting, than that queen-sized bed you still owe $212 on at Oak Street.

I. *You can do it all your life.* You might take a little longer, but if you think you're going to get off the hook by saying that you're over the hill sexually, you're wrong. While a quickie might be a misnomer for a seventy-year-old man, there's no question that a healthy, normal male can have sex for many more years.

IV. Metacare Planning Action Guidelines—For Better or Worse—Chapter 7

A. *How to develop companionship.* Mid-life is probably the first time since your honeymoon you can be companions. During the interim, your work and hers have often made that difficult at best. But now it's possible.

1. *Get acquainted first.* After a long absence or disengagement between partners, even for those who sleep together, it's important that they get reacquainted. Take her out to dinner; take her for walks. While getting reacquainted, talk generally about the present or the future, try not to go over all the problems of the past. Talking about the past is a typical cop-out in group counseling, so don't let that happen to you. Don't expect to become reacquainted too fast; give it some time.

2. *Look for the person inside your companion.* Try to stay away from talking about your role as the store manager or hers as mother. Stay away from subjects that you can hide behind. Ask questions about her.

3. *How to be friends—attempt to "peer" one another.* This is a technique used between equals and friends. When you talk to her, speak to her as a peer; don't talk down to her as a father would. "Peering" takes a little practice, particularly for the German commandant type or the "forty-year-old Daddy's little girl type. But you'll learn. You'll find it exciting and fun, as well as productive for your emerging personal relationship and growing companionship.

4. *Make other friends.* Make other friends *after* you've developed companionship with this significant other person. Don't escape from being friends with your wife by having dinner with the

gang or going to a church outing. Get acquainted
with each other without the neighborhood or the
family. It can be an exciting time for you. Then,
after you become comfortable with her, you
should venture out and renew yourself with
others.

5. *Friendship has no other goal.* Develop a companionship with her that does not always lead to sex
as a payoff. Sit around and smile at each other,
for example, but try not to have every instance of
companionship lead to the bed. This will reduce
sexual games and allow a genuine "I like you" to
build in their place.

B.   *Develop shared activities.* If you don't seem to have
anything in common, develop something.

1. Each of you should select an activity you've been
wanting to be involved in for some time. Describe the activity to the other and help him or
her get acquainted with it. You don't want
somebody just to go along for the ride; you want
somebody who can get involved with your activity, and vice-versa. These kinds of activities
are not easily developed. It takes two persons'
interest to build, not just one spectator and one
participant.

2. Make sure your new activities are selected to
allow each of you to grow in skill or knowledge
within the activity. One doesn't have to be the
professor and the other the student; each can
learn from the other.

3. Developing a separating activity. This sounds
like a contradiction, but it's important that men
and women have some separating activities as
well. You don't always have to have matching
bowling shirts. Do something without her, so you
have something to talk about other than bills and
back-porch repairs.

4. Don't develop too many activities. Some people

become so overladen with activities that they're unable to really be companions; they feel as though they have been on a grand tour of Europe for ten years. Rushing from one activity to another, from the beach to skydiving to boating to tennis, trying to get the most for your money, isn't going to help you develop companionship. Slow down. Be reasonable with your time and your money.

C. *How to be intimate.* Mid-life is an important time to develop intimacy.

1. Admit you need intimacy in this crazy, impersonal world. Go ahead, admit it! The kids on the playground won't call you a sissy.

2. Recognize that holding hands can be as important to you as an orgasm. Broaden your definition of intimacy. Don't feel you can solve all your closeness needs by a roll in the hay. Put sex in the proper perspective.

3. Select a second intimate place, other than the bedroom, a place where you can talk and hold each other. If you think this sounds funny, ask yourself what those who have affairs do.

4. Go away to the mountains or to the beach once every two or three months at least. If quarterly earnings affect your corporate life, just think what a quiet weekend alone together every three months might do for your marital life.

5. Learn to touch. If you want to learn to touch, you can. No one is going to tell you to keep your hands to yourself. Reach out and touch your partner. Try touching without words. Get used to communicating with each other through touching.

6. Give the other person unconditional love and closeness. Don't make her do something, whether it's cooking a good dinner or having a good time in bed, to get your love. Attempt to

develop what is called an unconditional love system, where you respect and love each other because—you love each other.

D. *Develop into a romantic.* It's surprising how most men feel about being romantic. The need for romance has no sexist characterists—ask a friend who's having an affair. Try to be more romantic if you haven't been before. It's amazing how writing in romantic terms can influence your observations and thinking about the world. Try writing your thoughts in a journal—thoughts of your partner, thoughts of your children. Write about nature, about your sexual encounters. Try drawing and painting as a way of developing your romantic characteristics. I know, you say you have absolutely no talent for art. Try it anyway. Everybody who observes can write or paint to some degree; everyone has some ability. One only needs enough gumption to risk his pen or brush.

Get away from thinking that a 20-minute sexual encounter is the only romantic act in life. Think about leading up to and following through on sexual activities. Your address and follow-through are important in golf—why not in sex as well?

Think of being a romantic in a larger picture. If you think a romantic is a sissy, be prepared to lose her to one. Remember, there's always a competitive market for an attractive woman.

E. *How to be exciting.* How can a middle-aged man be exciting? Well, certainly not by being a big drinker or acting out a delayed adolescence. If you were developing a new product line for your company, you'd work from the strengths of your previous product successes. Mid-life is your base upon which to be an exciting person. What can you offer that is exciting? Excitement has several properties:

1. It offers a change of pace, something unpredictable. Do something for and with her that is unorthodox, unprecedented, a change of pace.

2. The second property of excitement is emotional arousal. It can be stimulated by many things besides sexual foreplay. Try tickling her feet or taking her to a romantic French restaurant.

3. Involve yourself in activities that are exciting, such as backpacking or skiing.

4. Have a sense of adventure. Over and over again in middle-aged men's groups we find that men crave adventure—climbing mountains, buying a Maserati, or chasing young girls all are good examples. If what you need is adventure, build it into your new life. There are even raft trips down quiet rivers that you can enjoy with that important person in your life. Sporting activities such as sailing or skiing involve enough adventure for many metapausal men.

F. *Time requirements and "time for us."* This phrase from a popular song of the 1960s is not true of many relationships between a man and a woman. We tend to develop our companionship and relationships *after* all our time has been expended on other things.

1. Draw a pie chart showing how you spend an average day. See how much of your time is left for companionship (probably as little as ten minutes a day).

2. You must budget and calendar Metacare time for each other. Use your best calendaring techniques to cut out some time for "us." Mark it on your calendar if you need to.

3. Establish priorities for your time. Get some 3 x 5 cards and write down your major activities for the week, putting the approximate length of time each takes each week on the bottom of the card. Shuffle all the cards and then, sitting together with your partner, try to arrange a new priority system by placing the cards in the order you wish. This type of game is a spin-off of the in-basket game used by corporations, and it will

indicate how you want your time spent and how your time is actually spent.

G. *How to put some spirituality in your lives.* First, you must like yourself if you are going to love another. Second, you need to know how you and your relationships fit into the big picture of the universe. Consciously or unconsciously, we all have beliefs about how it all fits together, what life is all about, whether or not we believe in a Supreme Being. These important values are part of our sharing when we develop intimacy.

V. Metacare Action Planning Guidelines—Separating from Her—Chapter 8

Separation is probably one of the most reliable therapies for a conflicting marriage. Unfortunately, most feel that if they move out, it's all over. Not being at home causes the relationship to rupture further. While separation is difficult, it gives combatants time to ferret out issues and make decisions instead of those made after another marital "D day." Be careful you don't just use your separation as an excuse to goof around, though. Everyone gets manipulated then, including you.

A. *Knowing when you're trapped.* That you feel trapped is a figment of your imagination, a way to get off the hook, a way to justify your continued suffering. If you took this tack with your first client or customer, he would be your last. So admit to yourself that you don't have to suffer anymore, that you have the power to change where you are. In group counseling, we have noticed over and over again that many men who talk about the "I've-been-trapped" syndrome *really like it.* They bitch, but they like the security of being trapped. It's their rainy-day savings account. If this is true of you, try to make your marriage relationship the best one on the block, and then stop bellyaching. If you have tried to make your relationship work, without success, leave and find yourself another mate. There are many wonderful people around—you can do it. Unless illness or incredible circumstances prevent you, you are free to do what you want.

B. *Deciding if you can afford it.* This has been your excuse for a long time, hasn't it? Well, you can leave even if it means borrowing money for a while to get on your feet. You have borrowed for investments before in your life—isn't the investment in yourself worth it?

C. *Think of the children.* Would the kids be better off having a happy father whom they visit, or a miserable one at home? The latter alternative is a hell of a model for a kid to grow up with, isn't it?

D. *How not to be a blamer.* Don't continue to say that it's your wife's fault. The Blamer role doesn't suit you. It's just another one of your boyish tricks. If you want a mommy, stay where you are. But if you want to be a man, decide to love her or leave her.

E. *How to get trapped in an affair.* While some do carry on affairs that are undiscovered for years, for most the secret is short-lived, forcing those involved to make premature decisions. Remember that the tremendous freedom you feel you have with an affair can lead to another form of entrapment if you're discovered.

F. *Watch your divorce counseling.* If you contemplate a divorce, watch whom you talk to about it. Think through your confidant's motives for giving you advice. Your parents, a friend with a second wife, or a stick-to-itiveness type all have points of view that justify or protect their own position with the grand-kids or the new wife.

G. *How to mourn.* A divorce is a normal occasion for mourning. If you don't feel like going out during your mourning period, it's okay. Let that feeling take its course. It's crucial, however, to venture out after the mourning period is over. Start dating but don't merely bounce from one relationship into another; mourning is a poor reason to start another serious relationship. Try not to think yourself to death over a solution to your marital problems. For example, you may not be able to get a divorce and still have your children live with you. There may be no solution to some of your problems, but don't flagellate yourself over them. Take them one by one. You may overthink yourself into nonaction and be miserable all your life.

VI **Metacare Planning Guidelines—Who Calls the Shots—Chapter 9**
   A. *Deciding if you think you're better than she is.* Women's Liberation is here to stay: it's a viable and important concept that can't help but benefit the males in our society—if we can survive the transition. I'm talking about having a woman who can think, feel, and act independently without hanging all over you. So admit it's here to stay.
   B. *How not to get manipulated by the movement.* Several new manipulations are forcing themselves on many middle-aged men, causing many to resent the entire concept of Women's Liberation.
      1. Don't take on a new job around the house so that she can be liberated. You've already got enough work. If she has a full-time job, as you do, then get someone to help with the work at home, but don't add to your workaholic nature.
      2. Watch the money trip. Some women who are now working feel that whatever they make is their own. Either it's yours as well as hers, or yours isn't hers, either! On the other hand, don't take the money she earns and plunk it into something that only you want, like a boat, an airplane, or a sportscar. Learn how to share the decisions about spending income as well as making it.
      3. *Either she's independent or she isn't.* Don't baby

her one day to be completely dependent on you, and the next day, to be the first one on her block to head down Oak Street.

4. *Don't let her think that just because she's got a full-time job she's going to solve her identity problem.* While work is an important way for people to learn more about who they are, it certainly is not the complete answer. You've been working for twenty years and it hasn't done that much for you. Thousands of women are now taking full-time jobs in hopes that the purpose of their lives will suddenly become very clear. This, obviously, is impossible.

C. *Knowing about family adjustment.* Recognize that whether she goes to school or goes to work, *all members of the family will need to adjust* to this change. Don't tell her you think she should return to school or get a part-time job if you're going to get ticked off the first night you come home and your dinner isn't on the table.

D. *Preparing for the death of traditional male and female roles.* Don't go to war over who's the scientific one or whose role it is to mow the lawn as if your manhood is at stake.

E. *Be a person.* Define yourself as Joe or Sam or Jack, as she is trying to define herself as Sally or Mary. Be a person more than a set of roles. You'll find that you, too, can become liberated if you think as a person as well as the guy in the family with hair on his face.

F. *Knowing it's also difficult for the middle-aged woman.* It's hard for her to shift from being somebody's mother and doing housework to being a credit manager. You have difficult adjustments in your work; why shouldn't she in her work? Try to be understanding and help her grow more mature in her work. Your experience can be valuable to her. Many females know little about work. Help her!

G. *Understanding that menopause is a tough time for her, too.* Try not to let her excuse her lack of interest in you as a part of her change of life, and be careful yourself not to use metapause as your excuse for taking your secretary to lunch.

H. *Let her work and you stay home sometimes.* Let her do the bills and you do something else. Try to extend your partnership in marriage and add to its flexibility at the same time. You will find this rewarding for both of you.

VII. **Metacare Action Planning Guidelines—Has Anyone Seen My Father?—Chapter 10**

A. *Parents*

1. *How to look ahead.* Try to encourage your parents to keep looking ahead. Put some future in their lives. In old age, many parents become historians, constantly relating the past and ignoring the present or the future. This is a particularly difficult problem in our youth-oriented society.

2. *Keeping parents involved.* We've seen that one theory of aging is disengagement—that is, disengagement of older persons from friends and family activities. Keeping involved is clearly important. In California, for example, the average number of months that teachers receive retirement pay after retirement at the age of sixty-five, is eighteen months.[1] Sudden disengagement from their work might mean an earlier death for your parents. Plan ways you can involve your parents in your family life. Plan a scheduled event, part of a vacation, a weekend, or a Sunday dinner with them. Give them something to look forward to doing. Possibly you can plan a monthly schedule, for if they live only from day to day, they will have a greater chance of becoming disengaged. Planning and purpose

are important qualities of who we are at any age, including old age.

3. *Don't play father to your parents.* Many parents, as they age, tend to pick up dependency characteristics and childlike mannerisms. Don't let your parents force you into being *their* parents. Assist them; take care of them; but don't baby them. You will resent the extra father role being placed on you, and they will resent being treated like children. Moreover, don't cater to their every whim or ache and pain. Let them keep primary responsibility for themselves, if at all possible.

4. *How to watch your guilt.* Guilt is one of the most insidious things we deal with. Most middle-aged people have guilt feelings about their parents: "I don't spend enough time with them," "I should have been closer to my parents when they were more active." Much of this guilt develops when, as adolescents, we decide to separate ourselves from our parents. Being separated from your parents was critical for your own development. In those days, no matter what our parents said, we did the opposite, right? Now, when they have considerable leisure time, and you have as much responsibility as you'll ever carry, additional guilt seems to develop over how much attention you give them.

5. *Have several things they can do for you,* even if the events are not greatly important in your life. Parents get in the habit of doing things for their children; so, in later life, when there's nothing for them to do, relationship degeneration may occur more rapidly.

6. *How to have honest communication with your parents.* Make sure you communicate with your parents without always asking them how they are, as if you expected a catastrophe to befall them between phone calls. They pick up your

insecurities about them and apply them to themselves. Talk of things that you plan to do.

7. *Offer parents affection.* Love may be one of the strongest determinants of length of life; certainly you need to offer them your love. Forget about those early patterns of childhood when parents gave love and you accepted it. Reverse those patterns for a while.

8. *Life or death wish.* If you're like most men in our group-counseling sessions, you will discover two things about death. First, fear of death does not appear to be a major issue. Most men do not basically fear death, nor are they preoccupied with it in mid-life. Second, they wish to enjoy the rest of their lives to the utmost. This seems to be the major issue.

B. *Kids*

1. *Keep kids in the proper perspective.* Regardless of what people say, kids aren't more important than adults! True, they are important, they need more nurturing, more understanding, but they aren't more important. If you keep your children in perspective, you'll find that you won't resent them quite as much and their demands won't be burdensome. Other things and other persons are also important to you—admit it!

2. *Don't feel your children are rejecting you just because they need to pull away in adolescence.* It's normal, and you wouldn't have it any other way. You wouldn't want, at fifty, to be just like your father, would you?

3. *How to select a time and place.* Even though you live in the same house at the same time with your children, *don't feel that you live in the same time and place.* Values, forms of communication, and other differences between generations do exist; this does not mean that you need to be a member of the Pepsi Generation, and it doesn't mean that

your children always need to conform to the mores of the "father-knows-best" generation.

4. *Communication is more than just talking.* Listen to your kids. Select a time and place where you can talk over certain issues. Recognize the differences between you.

5. *Communication is respecting the person.* If you want to be respected as a person, *don't always play father,* because that's how you will get your respect—as Father, and not as Joe or Pete or Sam, the person.

These Metacare Guidelines should move the metapausal man from his itching to emansumation *if* he can do two things: look forward and plan for his future, and find the power to live that future.

Chapter 13

STEPPING INTO EMANSUMATION

We have found the metapausal man's identity slipping in many areas. The problem of The Gray Itch, the mid-life search for "me," threads through all the previous chapters. Sometimes laughing, sometimes serious, sometimes afraid, the middle-aged man moves through an unpredictable set of conditions beyond metapause.

"Let Me Out of Here" Summary

The typical man in mid-life is generally unaware of his own life cycle. He invests considerable time and effort in understanding Wall Street or judging the merchandise to buy for next summer's displays, but he doesn't know much about his own road ahead.

Just as he is unaware of his life cycle, he is equally unaware of the roles that he plays today. These roles wrap him in a cocoon of compacency until metapause. As district manager, daddy, or deacon, he moves through his twenties or thirties "becoming"—becoming what people expect him to be, or what he thinks he should be.

Then metathoughts begin cluttering his mind. He's confused in bed where it takes him longer to be aroused, or at work where he may find himself tired, bored, or even obsolete. He may be caught between generations. His usually predictable wife may go back to school or work. His secretary's legs may suddenly look very luscious to him. Collectively, these meta-thoughts spell out The Gray Itch.

Some men at this age knuckle under to what's "expected." Others choose to shed their roles and, like Gauguin, escape to a new world. Others don't consciously think about it, but they drink, screw, and hang-glide into later life. Like the fifty-five-year-old counselee who one night became impotent and the next day took up skydiving, many metapausal men simply do not know why they do things.

Take Roy, for example. Why would Roy, a person who's getting fatter and fatter by the day, buy sportcoats with larger and larger checks each month? Something must be operating, and that something is probably The Gray Itch.

Roy finds his career clock suddenly sticking or cuckooing constantly. He is fearful of becoming a cannonball salesman in 1980. Climbing up the ladder of his career, he reaches the ceiling. He suddenly asks, "Am I over the hill?" He wants to be his own boss, to have more control over his work. Yet, like many others, Roy barters these feelings for job security until retirement.

While the guys at the corner bar are still preoccupied with the sexual numbers game, Roy finds his sex life can't compete with the limericks and the war stories anymore. "They screwed for hours and hours, tore down trees, shrubs, and flowers" sounds like a fairy tale for adolescents. As his fears of sexual performance increase, he becomes more concerned with his "reviews" than with the performance itself, so he loses contact with his partner.

Other fears of sexual metapause occur, as a self-fulfilling prophecy develops.

Then Roy's parents age and pass away, a reminder that death is a reality, and that it will come to him, too. Undaunted, he's not really afraid of death, he just wants to make sure he lives the rest of his life.

Roy hides his boredom at work with more work—or forgets his family responsibilities with occasional irresponsibility.

He fails to see his changing silhouette through the flaked and chipped silver backing of the mirror of his past relationship with his wife. Roy finds that his wife walks with strides larger than his, meets the competition, and drinks ouzo straight these days. After twenty years of cooperation, how could she suddenly compete with him—doing her own thing?

Mirror after mirror, fogged by Roy's shortened breath or smudged by his unsure hands, indicates his increasing need to see clearly as he moves into the future. This could be a future where his confusion and suffering become a life-style—or a future where the awareness of metapause could become one of the most liberating discoveries of his life.

Emansumated Man

Unlike Roy, you have the opportunity to become an emansumated man. Emansumation is a coined word, our goal beyond metapause. It has three elements:

Emansumation is, first of all, an expression of *man*hood. Those of you who feel trapped, mere victims of circumstances, are risking a loss of your manhood. Where's your forcefulness, your power? In the old days, if there were no opportunities, you made them. When you had a point of view, you stuck with it. When you set a goal, you fought for it. Well, maybe it's time to get back some of these fiery definitions of manhood. You feel them smoldering in you, don't you? Are you worth it? Are you really trapped or have you merely been sitting with your legs crossed protecting your groin hoping for a miracle that will change your lot? Well, that's not going to happen. One of the most important aspects of mental health in middle age is *retaining control over our own lives.*

In group counseling, we have heard all the excuses: "I can't afford it," "It's too late," "Think of the kids." All have a discordant ring to them. You have one-third to one-half of your life remaining. You can wallow in your entrapment or move out briskly to live the "second half." You can ride it out—thirty more years full of ear horns, pacemakers, and flattened beer cans—or you can roar into your future in that new sportscar you always wanted—a future of power, opportunity, and love.

Furthermore, as an emansumated man, you have the opportunity to "throw up" that cynicism in you. You can substitute a new form of commitment and love. You may find you're more of a man than you thought. Leave the wham-banging to the so-called studs, counting up and bragging about their sources and their conquests, yet developing an increasing emptiness in their stomachs.

Emansumation is truly a redefinition of manliness; it's also a recognition that you are the sum total of your experience. Emansumation means you are the sum of who you are. When summing up, it's easy to see you are more than just your title in the company directory or a member of the Oak Street stop-sign committee. Sure, your kids need you, but you're more than just a father. Behind these giant roles, only partially seen, is the essential you. Discovery of this essential you may take some time or even some professional help, but you're there, alive and kicking. Bring that essential you forward; say excuse me to those crystallized roles you play, move to the front of the line!

Now look at mid-life. First, recognize you are in the middle of life; you're not the "Fonz," nor are you ready for the rest home. While you are changing, you can't erase your past or ignore your future. Experience counts in our society. Don't deny it; put it to work. Your past knowledge about your life can be turned into some wisdom. Your experience at work can be taught to younger colleagues. Your newfound self can be an exciting adventure.

If you look at yourself as the *sum* in eman*sum*ation, your before and after become pleasantly visible. The tumblers in the lock fall into place and that locked-up feeling is liberated. The days of being a spectator in your own life cycle are over. You are able to harmonize your life space as a total person beyond metapause.

Third, emansumation is also *emancipation.* We look around as we emerge from metapause, and clearly, we are free. Free to be who we are, free of the lofty expectations that we and others have of us. Free of being slaves to a twisted work ethic that measures manhood in terms of production units and sales quotas. Free of a body image unattainable by any but gifted decathlon stars. Free of clouded perceptions of love that center between our legs. Free of those tight-fitting roles that hamper us like a ten-dollar suit after a summer rain. Free of the cult of the young. Free to look at death, not out of fear, but in hopes of using the essential me for the rest of life.

The desire to be free, to be oneself, has preoccupied us for years. Suddenly it's here; we have it. We still fear freedom's partner, responsibility. However, the exciting discovery of the emansumated man is that freedom and responsibility are not opposites—one does not have to cast off his responsibilities to be free. One need only be responsible in the right areas. What is more emancipating than to know that you are free to choose to love someone else? How many restrictions, games, obligations, running-in-place activities disappear when we understand that freedom and responsibility are not opposites?

This is not a selfish, boastful sense of freedom and responsibility. It's a simple statement. If I'm responsible for myself, I'm also free to make choices—which, in turn, allow me the additional freedom to be responsible and love others.

Moving beyond metapause and curing The Gray Itch means becoming an emansumated man. Emansumation is manhood. Emansumation is the sum of your experiences as a total person. Emansumation is emancipation, freedom, and responsibility.

Power Source

Only one task remains: you need the power, the will to move beyond The Gray Itch, to stop scratching around, to set your sights to "go for it."

The power and the will to be an emansumated man in mid-life is probably our greatest definition of continuing manhood. It's easy to relinquish our power to others, to become passive, to allow our leverage to fade away. Most men, except those in the most adverse circumstances, have the power to be what they want to be in mid-life and after.

Whenever we wish to use one of our new gadgets or power tools, we must look for a power source or outlet. We would look

pretty silly standing with a new electric tool in our hand
without a power socket in sight. The same is true of emansumation. New insight, freedom, responsibility, and possibly even
manliness are in our hands, but we would look equally silly if
we were unable to find the power source to make these a
reality. Power sources to plug into are of two types, inside and
out, and both power sources work together.

Inside Power

Rule 1: *Admit you don't know yourself.* Inside power is the
most difficult to develop. Many middle-aged men refuse to look
at themselves, excusing their lack of care about themselves by
saying "I'm not a professional psychologist."

Rule 2: *Admit you have choices to make, that you're not
trapped.* One of the favorite metathoughts of metapausal men,
as we have seen, is "I'm trapped." On the contrary, you are
free.

Rule 3: *Set aside thirty minutes a week for you yourself.* Time
is a rare commodity. Most of us never seem to have time to
spend on ourselves. Well, you are quite good at scheduling your
work life. Buy some time for yourself, too.

Rule 4: *Don't fall for pat answers or extreme thinking about
male metapause.* We all want solutions to our problems with a
do-it-by-the-numbers approach. Unfortunately, The Gray Itch
doesn't have an easy cure. When I discuss male metapause with
friends, someone always says, "That's me—I have The Gray
Itch, but what is the answer?" While guidelines and hints can
be given, the mid-life male crisis is like adolescence in that the
problems adolescents have are not removed by a single
solution. Can you imagine someone asking, "What's the answer
to adolescence?"

Rule 5: *Emansumation must start with you being honest with
yourself.* Some men in group counseling are as afraid to talk to
themselves about their problems as they are to discuss them
with another. Many metapausal men who wish to think through
their problems using their inside power have no techniques for
doing it. One member of our counseling group, named Ralph,
asked, "What'll I do, sit under a tree and talk to myself?" The

answer to this question is a simple *yes!* It will not be easy at first. However, here are some techniques that may help you.

a. Keep a journal. Write down some of *your* feelings each week and examine them after a month.

b. Make a chart about your life with pros on one side and cons on the other.

c. Place some of your feelings on a cassette tape recorder and listen to them.

d. Make a priority pie; divide the pie into segments you desire, then compare them to the segments in your real "pie"— life. See any differences?

These are only a few rules and techniques for developing inside power to move beyond The Gray Itch to emansumated man.

The outside power you need can be supplied by many sources.

Outside Power

Rule 1: *Admit you could use someone to talk to about The Gray Itch.*

You need to find someone to talk to about metapause. Be willing to share yourself with another. You have talked for years to the bartender and barber about less significant things in your life.

Rule 2: *Follow the suggestions below in selecting a "friend" to talk to.* Whether the person you talk with is a man or woman is of little consequence. There are advantages in talking about certain subjects with either one or the other. Of all the outside sources that are possibilities, select one who has the following qualities:

a. Will keep his or her mouth shut.
b. Is probably not deeply associated with your work or family (unless a well-trusted member).
c. Is not going to lecture you.
d. Is not going to give you pat answers or judge the people involved.
e. Is willing to spend 70 percent of his or her own time

listening to you on this subject and not tell you his or her own story.

Rule 3: *Start by talking out your problem with your wife, but another person may be necessary.* The question always comes up: "Why shouldn't I talk to my wife about it?" The answer is, *do talk to her.* If you wish to develop intimacy and share your life with her, by all means tell her about your Gray Itch. However, if she has either been the cause of some of your problems or has been hurt by your "acting out" The Gray Itch, she may be less objective a person than you need to listen and help you.

Rule 4: *In looking for outside help, look for someone who can help you with a growth and development problem.* The Gray Itch can be an insignificant rash or a major medical and/or psychiatric problem. It is common and is not always defined as a "crisis." Therefore, don't be afraid to seek help from professionals. Generally, they and you should look at male metapause as a growth and development life stage and not as a terminal disease.

Rule 5: *Select someone, regardless of background, who can understand "where you're at."* Some say never go to a professional who is suffering from the same problem you are. Others believe your counselor must have gone through something like it if he is to help you. The answer here is that there is no answer. Select someone to help you *define* and develop outside power who has understanding of "where you're at." Other arguments are not very relevant.

Rule 6: *You don't have to go through The Gray Itch alone; there are many professionals, as well as friends, who can help you.* Any professional in the field of human behavior can help you. Physicians, teachers, college counselors, marriage and family counselors, ministers, and social workers can assist you, depending on the severity of your problem.

If you are apprehensive about going for professional counseling on a one-to-one basis, join one of the many male metapause groups forming throughout the country.

Inside and outside power development sources are many and

varied; try to develop both as far as possible and as needed. A few metapausal men think through this Gray Itch to become emansumated men by themselves; others will talk it through with a wife or friend; still others need themselves, family friends, and professional support.

Emansumated Man

Our purpose has been to expose The Gray Itch for what it is. We have also attempted to test where you are as a middle-aged man with the index of male metapause. Furthermore, we have made suggestions through Metacare Action Guidelines that will help you cope with your affliction. Lastly, we proposed a goal for those suffering from male metapause—that is, to move beyond it to emansumated manhood. Truly, a middle-aged man is the sum total of his experience, free to move ahead to discover and dominate it with his total person. His sources of power are many, as we have seen. Both inside and outside powers are available.

Now, good luck to you. You're likely to make your own good fortune if you bear in mind the sense of the quotation from Oliver Wendell Holmes with which this book began:

Life is action and passion: Therefore, it is required of a man that he should share the passion and action of his time at the peril of being judged not to have lived.

NOTES

Chapter 1

1. "Right or Left at Oak Street," Joe Nixon and Charlie Williams (Attache Music Publishers, Inc., 1969).

Chapter 3

1. Erik H. Erikson, *Childhood and Society,* 2nd ed. (New York: W. W. Norton and Co., 1963), pp. 247–268.
2. *Ibid.,* p. 249.
3. Douglas C. Kimmel, *Adulthood and Aging: An Interdisciplinary Approach* (New York: John Wiley and Sons, 1974), p. 24.
4. Erikson, p. 364.
5. Roger Gould, "Adult Life Stages: Growth Toward Self-Tolerance," *Psychology Today,* Feb. 1975, p. 74.
6. Robert C. Peck, "Psychological Developments in the Second Half of Life," in Bernice L. Neugarten, ed., *Middle Age and Aging* (Chicago: University of Chicago Press, 1968), pp. 89–90.
7. Erikson, p. 268.
8. Gould, p. 74.
9. Erikson, p. 268.

Chapter 4

1. "Second Acts in American Lives," *Time*, Mar. 8, 1968, p. 39.
2. Eleanor Fait, "Research Needs in Industrial Gerontology from Viewpoint of a State Employment Service," in Harold L. Sheppard, ed., *Toward an Industrial Gerontology* (Cambridge, Mass.: Schenkman Publishing Co., 1970), p. 90.
3. Cyril Sofer, *Men in Mid Career: A Study of British Managers and Technical Specialists* (Cambridge: Cambridge University Press, 1970), p. 92.
4. Douglas C. Kimmel, *Adulthood and Aging: An Interdisciplinary Approach* (New York: John Wiley and Sons, 1974), p. 243.
5. Kenneth Soddy and Mary C. Kidson, *Men in Middle Life* (London: Tavistock Publications, 1967), p. 345.
6. *Ibid.*, p. 118.
7. Sofer, p. 92.
8. U.S. Department of Labor, *The Pre-Retirement Years, Vol. 4. A Longitudinal Study of the Labor Market Experience of Men* (Washington: U.S. Government Printing Office, 1975), p. 3.
9. Dero A. Saunders, "Executive Discontent," in Sigmund Nosow and William H. Form, eds., *Man, Work and Society* (New York: Basic Books, Inc., 1962), p. 464.
10. R. Blauner, "Work Satisfaction and Industrial Trends in Modern Society," in W. Galenson and S. M. Lipset, eds., *Labor and Trade Unionism: An Interdisciplinary Reader* (New York: John Wiley and Sons, 1960), p. 89.
11. U.S. Department of Labor, pp. 120-122.
12. Sofer, p. 337.
13. Soddy and Kidson, p. 213.
14. Sofer, p. 272.
15. Studs Terkel, *Working-People Talk About What They Do All Day and How They Feel About What They Do* (New York: Avon Books, 1974), p. 531.
16. Terkel, pp. 436-437.

Chapter 5

1. Bernice L. Neugarten, "The Awareness of Middle Age," in *Middle Age and Aging* (Chicago: University of Chicago Press, 1968), pp. 93-98.
2. R. Hill and H. Montgomery, "Regional Changes and Changes Caused by Age in the Normal Skin," in Albert I. Lansing, ed., *Cowdrey's Problems of Aging—Biological and Medical Aspects,* 3rd ed. (Baltimore: The Williams and Wilkins Co., 1952), p. 769.
3. D. B. Bromley, *The Psychology of Human Aging,* 2nd ed. (Baltimore: Penguin Books, 1974), p. 86.
4. M. Prados and B. Ruddick, "Depressions and Anxiety States of the Middle-Aged Man," *The Psychiatric Quarterly* 21 (1947): pp. 410–430.
5. Estelle Ramey, "Men's Cycles," *Ms.,* Spring 1972, p. 11.
6. Kenneth Soddy and Mary C. Kidson, *Men in Middle Life* (London: Tavistock Publications, 1967), p. 97.
7. Peretz Lavie and Daniel F. Kripke, "Ultradian Rhythms: The 90-minute Clock Inside Us," *Psychology Today,* April 1975, p. 65.
8. Prados and Ruddick, p. 411.
9. William H. Masters and Virginia E. Johnson, *Human Sexual Response* (Boston: Little Brown and Co., 1966), p. 266.
10. H. L. Karpman and Sam Locke, *Your Second Chance* (Los Angeles: J. P. Tarcher, Inc., 1975), p. 183.
11. Paul B. Baltes and K. Warner Schaie, "Aging and I.Q.— The Myth of the Twilight Years," *Psychology Today,* March 1974, p. 38.
12. David Wechsler, *Manual for Adult Intelligence Scales— Tables 5 and 10* (New York: The Psychological Corporation, 1955).
13. Masters and Johnson, pp. 267–268
14. Paul D. White, "The Heart and Great Vessels in Old Age," in Albert I. Lansing, ed., *Cowdrey's Problems of Aging— Biological and Medical Aspects,* 3rd ed. (Baltimore: The William and Wilkins Co., 1952), p. 283.

15. Herbert Benson, *The Relaxation Response* (New York: William Morrow, Inc., 1975), p. 36.
16. T. H. Holmes and R. H. Rahe, "The Social Readjustment Rating Scale," *Journal of Psychosomatic Research* 11 (1967): 213–218.
17. Bromley, p. 243.

Chapter 6

1. William H. Masters and Virginia E. Johnson, *Human Sexual Inadequacy* (Boston: Little, Brown and Co., 1970), p. 159.
2. Myron Brenton, *The American Male* (Greenwich, Conn.: Fawcett Premier Books (1966), p. 159.
3. Fred Belliveau, *Understanding Human Sexual Inadequacy* (Boston: Little, Brown and Co., 1970), p. 102.
4. Herb Goldberg, *The Hazards of Being Male* (New York: Nash Publishing, 1976), p. 42.
5. Belliveau, p. 39.
6. Douglas C. Kimmel, *Adulthood and Aging: An Inter-disciplinary Approach* (New York: John Wiley and Sons, 1974), p. 147.
7. William H. Masters and Virginia E. Johnson, *Human Sexual Response* (Boston: Little Brown and Co., 1970), p. 270.
8. Belliveau, p. 213.
9. Belliveau, p. 113.
10. Helmut J. Ruebsaat and Raymond Hull, *The Male Climacteric* (New York: Hawthorn Books, Inc., 1975), p. 75.
11. Kimmel, p. 148.
12. Belliveau, p. 113.

Chapter 7

1. Douglas C. Kimmel, *Adulthood and Aging: An Inter-disciplinary Approach* (New York: John Wiley and Sons, 1974), p. 213.

2. James A. Peterson and Barbara Payne, *Love in the Later Years* (New York: Association Press, 1975), p. 24.
3. Kimmel, p. 215.
4. David Reuben, "The Marriage Game—How to Make the Magic Last," *Reader's Digest,* February 1976, p. 89.
5. Thelma C. Purtell, *Generation in the Middle* (New York: Paul S. Erikson, Inc., 1963), p. 83.
6. *Ibid.,* p. 88.
7. Eric Pfeiffer, Adriaan Verwoerdt, and Glenn C. Davis, "Sexual Behavior in Middle Life," *American Journal of Psychiatry* 128 (1972): 1262–1267.
8. Peter C. Pineo, "Disenchantment in the Later Years of Marriage," *Marriage and Family Living* 23 (1961): 3–11.
9. Myron Brenton, *The American Male* (Greewich, Conn.: Fawcett Premier Books, 1966), p. 94.

Chapter 8

1. James Kavanaugh, "To Begin to Live the Rest of My Life," in *There are Men too Gentle to Live Among Wolves* (New York: E. P. Dutton Co., 1970), p. 10.
2. Morton M. Hunt, *The World of the Formerly Married* (New York: McGraw-Hill Book Co., 1966), pp. 288–289.
3. Peter C. Pineo, "Disenchantment in the Later Years of Marriage," *Marriage and Family Living* 23 (1961): 3–11.
4. Alfred C. Kinsey, Wardell B. Pomeroy, Clyde E. Martin, and Paul H. Gebhard, *Sexual Behavior in the Human Female* (Philadelphia: W. B. Saunders Co., 1953), p. 433.
5. Morton Hunt, *The Affair* (New York: The World Publishing Co., 1969), p. 256.
6. Denis de Rougemont, *Love in the Western World,* rev. ed. (New York: Pantheon Books, 1956).
7. Philippe Ariès, "The Family Prison of Love," *Psychology Today,* Aug. 1975, p. 54.
8. Douglas C. Kimmel, *Adulthood and Aging: An Interdisciplinary Approach* (New York: John Wiley and Sons, 1974), p. 215.

9. Paul Bohannan, "The Six Stations of Divorce," in *Divorce and After* (Garden City: Doubleday and Co., 1970), pp. 29–55.

Chapter 9

1. Marc Feigen Fasteau, "The Male Machine—The High Price of Macho," *Psychology Today,* Sept. 1975, p. 60.
2. Herb Goldberg, *The Hazards of Being Male* (New York: Nash Publishing, 1976), p. 137.
3. Bernice L. Neugarten and Ruth J. Kraines, " 'Menopausal Symptoms' in Women of Various Ages," *Psychosomatic Medicine* 27 (1965): 266–273
4. *Ibid.,* p. 268.

Chapter 10

1. Margaret Mead, *Culture and Commitment—A Study of the Generation Gap* (Garden City, N.Y.: Doubleday and Co., Inc., 1970), p. 63.
2. C. P. Snow, source unknown.
3. Alvin Toffler, *Future Shock* (New York: Bantam Books, 1972), p. 83.
4. Edmond C. Hallberg and William G. Thomas, *When I Was Your Age—STOP* (New York: The Free Press, 1973), p. xvi.
5. Bernice L. Neugarten, "The Awareness of Middle Age," in *Middle Age and Aging* (Chicago: University of Chicago Press, 1968), pp. 93-98.
6. Kenneth Soddy and Mary C. Kidson, *Men in Middle Life* (London: Tavistock Publications, 1967), p. 215.

BIBLIOGRAPHY

Allport, G. W. *Pattern and Growth in Personality.* New York: Holt, 1961.

Anderson, P. B. "Women's Lib Drives Some Women to Psychiatrists." *The Los Angeles Times,* Jan. 4, 1976, p. 1.

Armstrong, J. R. and W. E. Tucker (eds.). *Injury in Sport.* Springfield, Ill.: Charles C. Thomas, 1964.

Arnstein, H. S. "The Crisis of Becoming a Father." *Sexual Behavior,* April 1972, pp. 42-47.

Bach, G. R. and H. Goldberg. *Creative Aggression.* Garden City, N.Y.: Doubleday & Co., 1974.

Baguedor, E. *Separation, Journal of a Marriage.* New York: Simon & Schuster, 1972.

Baltes, P. B. and K. W. Schaie. "Aging and I.Q.—The Myth of the Twilight Years." *Psychology Today* 7 (1974): 35-40

Bartolome, F. "Executives as Human Beings." *Harvard Business Review,* Nov.–Dec. 1972, pp. 62–69.

Belliveau, F. *Understanding Human Sexual Inadequacy.* Boston: Little, Brown and Co., 1970.

Benjamin, J. D. "Some Developmental Observations Relating to the Theory of Anxiety." *Journal of the American Psychoanalytic Association* 9 (1961): 652–68.

Benson, H. *The Relaxation Response.* New York: William Morrow and Co., Inc., 1975.

———. J. F. Beary, and M. P. Carol. "The Relaxation Response." *Psychiatry* 37 (1974): 37–46.

Bergler, E. *The Revolt of the Middle-Aged Man.* New York: Hill and Wang, Inc., 1957.

Bernard C. *Heart Attack: You Don't Have to Die.* New York: Delacorte, 1972.

Bernard, J. *The Future of Marriage.* New York: World Publishing Co., 1972.

Berne, E. *Games People Play.* New York: Grove Press, Inc., 1967.

Bettelheim, B. "The Problem of Generations." In E. H. Erikson (ed.), *The Challenge of Youth.* New York: Doubleday, 1963, pp. 77–109.

Bird, C. *Born Female.* New York: David McKay Co., Inc., 1968.

Bird, J., and L. Bird. *Marriage Is for Grownups.* Garden City, N.Y.: Doubleday and Co., Inc., 1969.

———.*Power to the Kids.* New York: Doubleday and Co., Inc., 1972.

Blauner, R. "Work Satisfaction and Industrial Trends in Modern Society." In W. Galenson and S. M. Lipset (eds.), *Labor and Trade Unionism: An Interdisciplinary Reader.* New York: John Wiley & Sons, 1960.

Blood, R. O. Jr., and D. M. Wolfe, *Husbands & Wives: The Dynamics of Married Living.* Glencoe, Ill.: The Free Press, 1964.

Blos, P. *On Adolescence: A Psychoanalytic Interpretation.* New York: Macmillan, 1961.

Bohannan, P. "The Six Stations of Divorce." In P. Bohannan (ed.), *Divorce and After.* Garden City, N.Y.: Doubleday and Co., 1970.

Bowlby, J. *Attachment and Loss.* Vol. 2, *Separation: Anxiety and Anger.* New York: Basic Books, 1973.

Brecher, R. and E. (eds.). *An Analysis of Human Sexual Response.* New York: New American Library, Signet Books, 1966.

Brenton, M. *The American Male.* Greenwich, Conn.: Fawcett Publications, Inc., 1966.

———.*Sex and Your Heart.* New York: Coward-McCann, 1968.

"The Broken Family: Divorce U.S. Style." *Newsweek,* Mar. 12, 1973, pp. 45–57.

Bromley, D. B. *The Psychology of Human Aging.* 2nd ed. Baltimore: Penguin Books, Inc., 1974.

Brooks, R. and J. Poe. Screenplay of *Cat on a Hot Tin Roof* by Tennessee Williams, an Avon Production for Metro-Goldwyn-Mayer, 1959.

Brown, M. "Keeping Marriage Alive" *McCalls,* Jan. 1973.

Burgess, E. W., and L. S. Cottrell, Jr. *Predicting Success or Failure in Marriage.* New York: Prentice-Hall, Inc., 1939.

Burr, W. R. "Satisfaction with Various Aspects of Marriage over the Life Cycle: A Random Middle Class Sample." *Journal of Marriage and the Family* 32 (1970): 29–37.

Cabot, N. H. *You Can't Count on Dying.* Boston: Houghton Mifflin, Inc., 1961.

Campbell, A. "The American Way of Mating: Marriage Si, Children Only Maybe." *Psychology Today* 8 (1975): 37–43.

Casady, M. "Runaway Wives: Husbands Don't Pick Up the Danger Signals Their Wives Send Out. *Psychology Today* 8 (1975): 42.

Center for the Study of Higher Education. *Omnibus Personality Inventory Research Manual.* Berkeley: University of California, 1964.

Chew, P. *The Inner World of the Middle-Aged Man.* New York: Macmillan Publishing Co., 1976.

Cimons, M. "American Women Forgotten at Forty?" *Los Angeles Times, View,* Mar. 16, 1975.

Collier, M. J., and E. L. Gaier. "The Hero in the Preferred Childhood Stories of College Men. *American Image* 16 (1956): 177–194.

Crystal, J. C., and R. N. Bolles. *Where Do I Go From Here with My Life?* New York: The Seabury Press, 1974.

Curran, J. P. *Primer of Sports Injuries.* Springfield, Ill.: Charles C. Thomas, 1968.

Davis, J. *Great Aspirations: The Graduate School Plans of America's College Seniors.* Chicago: Aldine, 1964.

Davis, R. (ed.). *Aging: Prospects and Issues.* A monograph from the Ethel Percy Andrus Gerontology Center, University of Southern California, Los Angeles, 1973.

Davitz, J. and L. Davitz. *Making It from 40 to 50.* New York: Random House, 1976.

de Rougemont, D. *Love in the Western World.* New York: Pantheon Publishing Co., 1956.

Deutsch, H. *The Psychology of Women.* New York: Grune & Stratton, 1944.

Development and Aging. Washington, D.C.: The American Psychological Association, 1973.

Eliade, M. *Yoga: Immortality and Freedom.* Trans. W. R. Trask. London: Routledge and Kegan Paul, 1958.

Elkisch, P. "The Psychological Significance of the Mirror." *Journal of the American Psychoanalytic Association* 5 (1957): 235–244.

Entine, A. (ed.). *Americans in Middle Years: Career Options and Educational Opportunitues.* Los Angeles: Ethel Percy Andrus Gerontology Center, 1974.

Erikson, E. H. *Childhood and Society.* 2nd ed. New York: Norton, 1963.

———. "Growth and Crises of the Healthy Personality." *Psychological Issues* 1 (1959): 98.

———. *Identity and the Life Cycle.* New York: International Universities Press, 1959.

———. *Identity: Youth and Crisis.* New York: Norton, 1968.

Fannin, L. F., and M. B. Clinard. Difference in the conception of self as a male among lower and middle class delinquents. *Social Problems,* 1966, 13, 205-214.

Farnsworth, D. "A Psychiatrist Reflects on College Education." Address at Jesuit Educational Association, Chicago, Apr. 11, 1966.

Farrell, B. "You've Come a Long Way, Buddy." *Life,* Aug. 27, 1971, p. 51.

Farrell, W. *The Liberated Man—Beyond Masculinity: Freeing Men and Their Relationships with Women.* New York: Random House, 1974.

Fasteau, M. *The Male Machine.* New York: Delta Publishing Co., 1976.

———. "The Male Machine—the High Price of Macho." *Psychology Today* 9 (1975): 60.

Feldman, K. S., and T. M. Newcomb. *The Impact of College on Students.* San Francisco: Jossey-Bass, 1969.

Fenichel, O. "Identification." In *The Collected Papers of Otto Fenchel.* Vol. 1. New York: Norton, 1953, pp. 97–113.

——. *The Psychoanalytic Theory of Neurosis.* New York: Norton, 1945.

Feshbach, S., and N. Feshbach, "The Young Aggressors." *Psychological Monographs,* 81 (1970): 132–142.

Fischer, P. *The Gay Mystique.* New York: Stein & Day, 1972.

Forsyth, R. P. "Blood Pressure and Avoidance Conditioning: A Study of 15-day Trials in the Rhesus Monkey. *Psychosomatic Medicine* 30 (1968): 125–135.

Frankel, C. "The Third Great Revolution of Mankind." *The New York Times Magazine,* Feb. 9, 1958.

Freedman, M. B. "Studies of College Alumni." In N. Sanford (ed.), *The American College.* New York: Wiley, 1962, pp. 847–886.

Freud, A. "The Ego and the Mechanisms of Defense." In *The Writings of Anna Freud.* Vol. II. New York: International Universities Press, 1936.

Freud, S. *Beyond the Pleasure Principle,* 1920. Standard Edition, Vol. XVIII. London: Hogarth Press, 1955.

——. *The Interpretation of Dreams,* 1900. Standard Edition, Vols. IV, V. London: Hogarth Press, 1966.

——. *Mourning and Melancholia,* 1917. Standard Edition, Vol. XIV. London: Hogarth Press, 1957.

Fried, B. *The Middle Age Crisis.* New York: Harper and Row, Inc., 1967.

Friedenberg, E. Z. *The Vanishing Adolescent.* Boston: Beacon Press, 1959.

Friedman, M., and R. H. Rosenman. "Association of Specific Overt Behavior Pattern with Blood and Cardiovascular Findings." *Journal of the American Medical Association,* 169 (1959): 1286–1296.

Fromm, E. *The Art of Loving.* New York: Harper & Bros., 1956.

Fromm-Reichmann, F. "On Loneliness." In D. M. Bullard (ed.), *Selected Papers of Frieda Fromm-Reichmann.* Chicago: University of Chicago Press, 1959, pp. 325–336.

Furer, M. "The History of the Superego Concept in Psychoanalysis: A Review of the Literature. In S. C. Post (ed.), *Moral Values and Superego Concept in Psychoanalysis.* New York: International Universities Press, 1972, pp. 11–63.

Galbraith, J. K. *The Affluent Society.* New York: New American Library, 1958.

Gergen, K. J. *The Concept of Self.* New York: Holt, Rinehart & Winston, 1971.

Gewirtz, J. L. (ed.). *Attachment and Dependency.* Washington, D.C.: V. H. Winston & Sons, 1972.

"Girlish Boys." Time, Nov. 26, 1973, p. 33.

Goffman, E. *The Presentation of Self in Everyday Life.* Garden City, N.Y.: Doubleday, Anchor, 1959.

Goldberg, H. *The Hazards of Being Male.* New York: Nash Publishing, 1976.

Goldfried, M. R. and M. Merbaum. "How to Control Yourself." *Psychology Today* 7 (1973): 102–104.

Goode, W. J. *After Divorce.* New York: The Free Press, 1956.

Gordon, C., C. M. Graitz, and J. Scott. "Value Priorities and Leisure Activities Among Middle Aged and Older Anglos." *Diseases of the Nervous System* 34 (1973): 13–26.

Gould, R. "Adult Life Stages: Growth toward self-tolerance." *Psychology Today,* 8 (1975): 74–78.

———.*Child Studies Through Fantasy: Cognitive-Affective Patterns in Development.* New York: Quadrangle Books, 1972.

———."The Phases of Adult Life: A Study in Developmental Psychology." *The American Journal of Psychology* 129 (1972): 33–43.

Gove, W. R. "The Relationship Between Sex Roles, Marital Status, and Mental Illness. *Social Forces,* Sept. 1972, pp. 34–44.

Greenleigh, L. "Facing the Challenge of Change in Middle Age." *Geriatrics* 29 (1974): 61–68.

Gronseth, E. "The Breadwinner Trap." In L. Howe (ed.), *The Future of the Family.* New York: Simon & Schuster, 1972, pp. 175–191.

Gunther, M. "The Female Fears That Bind a Man." *True,* Feb. 1965.

Hallberg, E. C., and W. G. Thomas. *When I Was Your Age—*

STOP. New York: The Free Press, 1973.

Hannah, W. *Differences Between Drop-outs and Stay-ins at Entrance—1965 Freshman.* Paper presented at the 1967 Workshop on Student Development in Small Colleges, Racine, Wis., Aug. 1967.

Hapgood, D. *The Screwing of the Average Man.* New York: Doubleday, Inc., 1975.

Hare, N. "The Frustrated Masculinity of the Negro Male." In R. Staples (ed.), *The Black Family: Essays and Studies.* Belmont, Calif.: Wadsworth, 1971, pp. 131–134.

Harlow, H. F. "The Nature of Love." *American Psychologist* 13 (1958): 673–685.

Harris, J. *The Prime of Ms America.* New York: G. P. Putnam's Sons, 1975.

Harris, T. A. *I'm OK, You're OK.* New York: Avon Books, 1969.

Heidegger, M. *Being and Time.* New York: Harper & Row, 1962.

Heist, P. (ed.). *The Creative College Student: An Unmet Challenge.* San Francisco: Jossey-Bass, 1968.

Hodges, P. "The Male Mastectomy." *Moneysworth* 13 (1975): 8–10.

Holmes, T. H., and M. Masuda. "Psychosomatic Syndrome." *Psychology Today* 5 (1972): 71–72, 106.

Holmes, T. H. and R. H. Rahe. "The Social Readjustment Rating Scale." *Journal of Psychosomatic Research* 11 (1967): 213.

Horn, J. "Happiness Is . . . an Empty Nest." *Psychology Today* 9 (1976): 22.

Hunt, M. *The World of the Formerly Married.* New York: McGraw-Hill, 1966.

Huxley, J. *Man in the Modern World.* New York: Mentor Books (The New American Library), 1944.

Huyck, M. H. *Growing Older.* Englewood Cliffs, N.J.: Prentice Hall, Inc., 1974.

Ismail, A. H., and L. E. Trachtman. "Jogging the Imagination." *Psychology Today* 6 (1973): 79–82.

Jackard, C. R., Jr. "The American Male Rejects Counseling."

Adult Leadership, May 1974, pp. 9–10, 32.

———. Jacobson, E. Progressive Relaxation. Chicago: University of Chicago Press, 1938.

Jourard, S. "Some Lethal Aspects of the Male Role." Chap. 6 of *The Transparent Self.* Princeton, N.J.: Van Nostrand, 1964, pp. 46–55.

———. *The Transparent Self.* Rev. Ed. Princeton, N.J.: Van Nostrand Co., 1971, p. 40.

Kalish, R. A. "The Effects of Death upon the Family." In L. Pearson (ed.), *Death and Dying.* Cleveland and London: The Press of Western Reserve University, 1969.

Karpman, H. L., and S. Locke. *Your Second Life.* Los Angeles: J. P. Tarcher, Inc., 1975.

Keniston, K. "Social Change and Youth in America." In E. H. Erikson (ed.), *The Challenge of Youth.* New York: Doubleday, 1965, pp. 191–222.

Kimmel, D. C. *Adulthood and Aging: An Interdisciplinary Approach.* New York: John Wiley & Sons, 1974.

Kinsey, A. C., W. B. Pomeroy, and C. E. Martin. *Sexual Behavior in the Human Male.* 2d ed. Philadelphia: Saunders, 1953.

Kinsey, A. C., W. B. Pomeroy, C. E. Martin, and P. H. Gebhard. *Sexual Behavior in the Human Female.* Philadelphia: W. B. Saunders Co., 1953.

Klopfer, P. H., D. K. Adams, and M. S. Klopfer. "Mother Love: What Turns It On?" *American Science* 59 (1971): 404–407.

Komarovsky, M. *Blue-Collar Marriage.* New York: Vintage Books, 1967.

———. *The Unemployed Man and His Family.* New York: Institute of Social Research, 1940.

———. *Women in the Modern World.* Boston: Little Brown & Co., 1953.

Korda, M. *Male Chauvinism: How It Works.* New York: Random House, 1973.

Kraines, R. "The Menopause and Evaluation of the Self: A Study of Women in the Climacteric Years." Unpublished doctoral dissertation, University of Chicago, Committee on Human Development, 1963.

Kübler-Ross, E. *On Death and Dying.* New York: The Macmillan Co., 1969.

Lannholm, G. V., and B. Pitcher. *Mean Score Changes on the Graduate Record Examinations Area Tests for College Students Tested Three Times in a Four Year Period.* Princeton, N.J.: Educational Testing Service, 1959.

Lansing, A. I. (ed.). *Cowdrey's Problems of Aging—Biological and Medical Aspects.* 3d ed. Baltimore: The Williams and Wilkins Co., 1952.

Lavie, P. and D. F. Kripke. "Ultradian Rhythms: The 90-Minute Clock Inside Us." *Psychology Today* 8 (1975): 54–65.

Le Shan, E. *The Wonderful Crisis of Middle Age.* New York: David McKay, 1973.

Lear, M. W. "Is There a Male Menopause?" *The New York Times Magazine,* Jan. 28, 1973.

Lennon, J. and P. McCartney. "When I'm Sixty-four." Copyright by Northern Songs, Ltd., 1967.

Levine, S. "One Man's Experience." *MS,* Feb. 1973, p. 14.

Levinson, D. "The Male Mid-life Decade." In D. Ricks (ed.), *Life History Research in Psychopathology.* Vol. II. Minneapolis: University of Minnesota Press, 1974.

———. "The Psychological Development of Men in Early Adulthood and the Mid-life Transition." Minneapolis: University of Minnesota Press, 1974.

Levinson, H. "On Being a Middle-Aged Manager." *Harvard Business Review,* July–August, 1969.

Levy, D. M. *Maternal Overprotection.* New York: Columbia University Press, 1943.

Lieberman, M. A., and A. S. Coplan. "Distance from Death as a Variable in the Study of Aging." *Developmental Psychology* 2 (1970): 71–84.

Lincoln. M. *Your Health, Sir!* New York: Harper & Bros., 1953.

Livesay, T. M. "Does Intelligence Increase at the College Level?" *Journal of Educational Psychology,* 30 (1939): 63–68.

Lowenthal, M.F., and D. Chiriboga. "Transition to the Empty Nest." *Archives of General Psychiatry,* 26.

Luce, G. G. "Trust Your Body Rhythms." *Psychology Today,* 8 (1975): 52–53.

Lynd, H. M. *On Shame and the Search for Identity.* New York: Harcourt, Brace, 1958.

Maccoby, E. (ed.). *The Development of Sex Differences.* Stanford, Calif.: Stanford Universtiy Press, 1966.

Macleish, A. "The Great American Frustration." *Saturday Review,* July 13, 1968.

Marmor, J. *Sexual Inversion: The Multiple Roots of Homosexuality.* New York: Basic Books, 1965.

Masters, W. H., and V. E. Johnson. *Human Sexual Inadequacy.* Boston: Little, Brown & Co., 1970.

———.*Human Sexual Response.* Boston: Little, Brown & Co., 1966.

May, R. *Love and Will.* New York: Norton, 1969.

McKain, W. *Retirement Marriage.* Storrs, Conn.: Storrs Agricultural Experiment Station Monograph 3, 1969.

McLuhan, M. and Q. Fiore. *The Medium Is the Message.* New York: Bantam Books, 1967.

Mead, G. H. *Mind, Self and Society.* Chicago: University of Chicago Press, 1934.

Mead, M. *Blackberry Winter: My Earlier Years.* New York: William Morrow, 1972.

———. *Culture and Commitment—A Study of the Generation Gap.* Garden City, N.Y.: Doubleday and Co., Inc, 1970.

———. *Male and Female.* New York: William Morrow & Co., 1949.

———. Sex and Temperament in Three Primitive Societies. New York: William Morrow & Co., 1935.

Morgan, M. *The Total Woman.* Old Tappan, N.J.: Fleming H. Revell, 1973.

Mousseau, J. "The Family, Prison of Love." *Psychology Today,* 9 (1975): 52–58.

Moustakas, C. E. *Loneliness.* Englewood Cliffs, N.J.: Prentice-Hall, Inc., 1961.

Murphy, G. *Human Potentialities.* New York: Basic Books, 1958.

Neugarten, B. L. "Dynamics of Transition of Middle Age to Old Age—Adaptation of the Life Cycle." *Journal of Geriatric Psychiatry* 4 (1970): 71–100.

———. "Grow Old along with Me! The Best Is Yet to Be." *Psychology Today* 5 (1971): 45–48, 79–81.

———. *Middle Age and Aging: A Reader in Social Psychology.* Chicago: University of Chicago Press, 1968.

———. "Summary and Implications." In B. L. Neugarten and Associates, *Personality in Middle and Late Life.* New York: Atherton Press, 1964, pp. 188–200.

———, and N. Datan. "The middle years." In S. Arieti (ed.), *American Handbook of Psychiatry.* Vol. 1. New York: Basic Books, Inc., 1974.

———.R.J. Kraines. "Menopausal Symptoms in Women of Various Ages." Psychosomatic Medicine 27 (1965): 266–273.

———, and D. C. Garron. "Attitudes of Middle-aged Persons Toward Growing Old. *Geriatrics* 14 (1959): 21–24.

———, V. Wood, R. Kraines, and B. Loomis. "Women's Attitudes Toward the Menopause." *Vita Humana* 6 (1963): 140–51.

Newcomb, T. M. *Personality and Social Change.* New York: Dryden Press, 1943.

Nydegger, C. "The Older the Father: Late Is Great." *Psychology Today,* Apr. 1974, pp. 26–28.

O'Neill, N. and G. O'Neill. *Open Marriage.* New York: Avon Books, 1973.

———. *Shifting Gears.* New York: Avon Books, 1974.

Patel, C. H. "Yoga and Biofeedback in the Management of Hypertension. *Lancet* ii (1973): 1053–1055.

Paul, J. and M. *Free to Love.* Los Angeles: J. P. Tarcher, Inc., 1975.

Peterson, J. A. *Married Love in the Middle Years.* New York: Association Press, 1968.

———, and B. Payne. *Love in the Later Years.* New York: Association Press, 1975.

Piaget, J. *The Construction of Reality in the Child.* New York: Basic Books, 1954.

———. *Play, Dreams and Imitation in Childhood.* New York: Norton, 1962.

Pineo, P. C. "Disenchantment in the Later Years of Marriage." *Marriage and Family Living* 23 (1961): 3–11

Pincus, L. *Death and the Family.* New York: Pantheon Books, 1974.

Playboy panel: The Womanization of America." *Playboy,* June 1962.

Pleck, J. and J. Sawyer (eds.). *Men and Masculinity.* New York: Prentice-Hall Spectrum Books, 1974.

Purtell, T. C. *Generation in the Middle.* New York: Paul S. Erikson, Inc., 1963.

Ramey, E. "A Feminist Talks to Men." *John Hopkins Magazine,* Sept. 1973.

——. "Men's Cycles." *Ms.,* Spring 1972. pp. 8ff.

Rapoport, R. N. *Mid-Career Development.* London: Tavistock Publications, 1970.

Riesman, D. "Permissiveness and Sex Roles." *Marriage and Family Living,* Aug. 1959.

Riley, M. W., M. Johnson, and A. Foner. *Aging and Society. Vol. 3: A Sociology of Age Stratification.* New York: Russell Sage Foundation, 1972.

Rogers, C. *Becoming Partners: Marriage and Its Alternatives.* New York: Delacorte Press, 1972.

——. *On Becoming a Person.* Boston: Houghton Mifflin, 1961.

Rollins, B. C., and H. Feldman. "Marital Satisfaction over the Family Life Cycle." *Journal of Marriage and the Family* 32 (1970): 20–28.

Reubsaat, H. J., and R. Hull. *The Male Climacteric.* New York: Hawthorn Books, 1975.

Saunders, D. A. "Executive Discontent." In S. Nosow and W. H. Form (eds.), *Man, Work and Society.* New York: Basic Books, 1962, pp. 461–467.

Sawyer, J. "On Male Liberation." *Liberation* 15 (1970): 6–8.

——. "On the Politics of Male Liberation. *Win* 8 (1971): 20–21.

Saxe, L. P., and N. B. Garson. *Sex and the Mature Man.* New York: Gilbert Press, Inc., 1964.

Schoenberg, J. and J. Stichman. *How to Survive Your Husband's Heart Attack.* New York: David McKay, 1974.

Scott, J. "It's Not How You Play the Game, but What Pill You Take." *New York Times Magazine,* Oct. 17, 1971, pp. 40–41.

Sears, R. R., and S. S. Feldman (eds.). *The Seven Ages of Man.*

Los Altos, Calif.: William Kaufman, 1973.

"Second Acts in American Lives." *Time,* Mar. 8, 1968, p. 39.

Sheehy, G. "Can Couples Survive?" *New York,* Feb. 19, 1973.

——. "Catch-30 and Other Predictable Crises of Growing Up Adult." *New York,* Feb. 18, 1974.

——. "Mid-life Crisis: Best Chance for Couples to Grow Up." *New York,* Apr. 29, 1974.

——. "The Sexual Diamond: Facing the Facts of the Male and Female Sexual Life Cycles." *New York,* Jan. 26, 1976.

——. *Passages—Predictable Crisis of Adult Life.* New York: E. P. Dutton and Co., Inc., 1976.

Shostak, A. B. "Middle-aged Working Class Americans at Home." *Occupational Mental Health* 2 (1972): 2–7.

Smith, M. B. "Personal Values in the Study of Lives." In R. W. White (ed.), *The Study of Lives.* New York: Atherton Press, 1963, pp. 324–347.

Soddy, K., and M. C. Kidson. *Men in Middle Life.* Philadelphia: J. B. Lippincott, 1967.

Sofer, C. *Men in Mid Career: A Study of British Managers and Technical Specialists.* Cambridge: Cambridge University Press, 1970.

Steiner, R. "The Sacred Bull: A Bibliography on Male Birth Control." *Synergy* 40 (1973).

Steinmann, A., and D. J. Fox. *The Male Dilemma.* New York: Jason Aronson, 1973.

Stetson, D. *Starting Over.* New York: The Macmillan Co., 1971.

Sugarman, D. A. "Male Impotence: What Every Woman Should Know." *Reader's Digest,* Sept. 1973, pp. 91–95.

Terkel, S. *Working People Talk about What They Do All Day and How They Feel about What They Do.* New York: Avon Books, 1974.

Thoreau, H. D. *Walden.* Columbus, Ohio: Charles E. Merrill Publishing Co., 1969.

Tiger, L. "A Rugged Road for Executives Who Get Married." *Los Angeles Times,* Sept. 22, 1974, pp. 1, 12.

Toffler, A., *Future Shock.* New York: Random House, 1970.

U. S. Department of Health, Education, and Welfare. "Marriage Statistics, 1969, and Births, Marriages, Divorces, and Deaths for 1973." *Vital Statistics Report,* 1969.

U.S. Department of Labor. *The Pre-Retirement Years. Vol. 4: A Longitudinal Study of the Labor Market Experience of Men.* Washington, D.C.: U.S. Government Printing Office, 1975.

Useem, R. H., et al. "The Function of Neighboring for the Middle-Class Male." *Human Organization* 19 (1960): 68–76.

Vedder, C. B. (ed.). *Problems of the Middle-Aged.* Springfield, Ill.: Charles C. Thomas, 1965.

Vils, U. "Changing Careers in Midstream." *Los Angeles Times,* July 18, 1975, pp. 1, 8.

Wheelis, A. *The Quest for Identity.* New York: W. W. Norton, 1958.

Wills, G. "What? What? Are Young Americans Afraid to Have Kids?" *Esquire,* Mar. 1974.

Winter, R. "Biological Superiority—Female or Male." *Science Digest,* Aug. 1971, p. 50.

Wolfe, L. *Playing Around.* New York: William Morrow, 1975.

INDEX